to

my beloved family

CBS Confident Pharmacy Series

Hospital and Clinical Pharmacy

Third Edition

for Second Year Diploma in Pharmacy

(**0816**) Strictly Based on Syllabus as per ER1991

Question–Answer Type Notes and Board Question Papers (1996 to 2017)

Salient Features

- Total Confidence and 100 percent Success in Every Examination.
- Repeatedly Asked Board Questions Indicated in Brackets.
- Chapterwise Collection of Very Important Questions.
- Written in Very Simple and Lucid Language.
- Board Question Papers 2015–2017 given at the End of Text.

CBS Titles by the same Author in

CBS Confident Pharmacy Series

First Year D Pharm

1. Pharmaceutics I, 3/e
2. Pharmaceutical Chemistry I, 3/e
3. Pharmacognosy, 3/e
4. Biochemistry and Clinical Pathology, 3/e
5. Human Anatomy and Physiology, 3/e
6. Health Education and Community Pharmacy, 3/e

Second Year D Pharm

1. Pharmaceutics II, 3/e
2. Pharmaceutical Chemistry II, 3/e
3. Pharmacology and Toxicology, 3/e
4. Pharmaceutical Jurisprudence, 3/e
5. Drug Store and Business Management, 3/e
6. Hospital and Clinical Pharmacy, 3/e

CBS Confident Pharmacy Series

Hospital and Clinical Pharmacy

Third Edition

for Second Year Diploma in Pharmacy

(**0816**) Strictly Based on Syllabus as per ER1991

V.N. Raje M Pharm

Principal
Gourishankar Education Society's
GES College of Pharmacy (D Pharm)
Limb, Satara, Maharashtra

CBS

CBS Publishers & Distributors Pvt Ltd

New Delhi • Bengaluru • Chennai • Kochi • Kolkata • Mumbai
Hyderabad • Jharkhand • Nagpur • Patna • Pune • Uttarakhand

Disclaimer

Science and technology are constantly changing fields. New research and experience broaden the scope of information and knowledge. The author has tried his best in giving information available to him while preparing the material for this book. Although, all efforts have been made to ensure optimum accuracy of the material, yet it is quite possible some errors might have been left uncorrected. The publisher, the printer and the author will not be held responsible for any inadvertent errors or inaccuracies.

Hospital and Clinical Pharmacy
Third Edition

ISBN: 978-93-86478-49-8

Third Edition: 2018
Reprint: 2018, 2019
First Edition: 2010
Reprint: 2011
Second Edition: 2015
Reprint: 2016

Published by Satish Kumar Jain and produced by Varun Jain for
CBS Publishers & Distributors Pvt Ltd
4819/XI Prahlad Street, 24 Ansari Road, Daryaganj, New Delhi 110 002, India.
Ph: 23289259, 23266861, 23266867 Website: www.cbspd.com
Fax: 011-23243014 e-mail: delhi@cbspd.com; cbspubs@airtelmail.in.
Corporate Office: 204 FIE, Industrial Area, Patparganj, Delhi 110 092
Ph: 4934 4934 Fax: 4934 4935 e-mail: publishing@cbspd.com; publicity@cbspd.com

Branches

- **Bengaluru:** Seema House 2975, 17th Cross, K.R. Road, Banasankari 2nd Stage, Bengaluru 560 070, Karnataka
  Ph: +91-80-26771678/79 Fax: +91-80-26771680 e-mail: bangalore@cbspd.com
- **Chennai:** 7, Subbaraya Street, Shenoy Nagar, Chennai 600 030, Tamil Nadu
  Ph: +91-44-26680620, 26681266 Fax: +91-44-42032115 e-mail: chennai@cbspd.com
- **Kochi:** Ashana House, No. 39/1904, AM Thomas Road, Valanjambalam, Ernakulam 682 016, Kochi, Kerala
  Ph: +91-484-4059061-65 Fax: +91-484-4059065 e-mail: kochi@cbspd.com
- **Kolkata:** 6/B, Ground Floor, Rameswar Shaw Road, Kolkata-700 014, West Bengal
  Ph: +91-33-22891126, 22891127, 22891128 e-mail: kolkata@cbspd.com
- **Mumbai:** 83-C, Dr E Moses Road, Worli, Mumbai-400018, Maharashtra
  Ph: +91-22-24902340/41 Fax: +91-22-24902342 e-mail: mumbai@cbspd.com

Representatives

• **Hyderabad**	0-9885175004	• **Jharkhand**	0-9811541605	• **Nagpur**	0-9021734563
• **Patna**	0-9334159340	• **Pune**	0-9623451994	• **Uttarakhand**	0-9716462459

Printed at Mudrak, Noida, UP, India

Preface to the Third Edition

The third edition of the now popular and successful book includes Board Question Papers 1996 to 2017. The book has been written to meet the requirements of students of Diploma in Pharmacy (D Pharm) in accordance with the new revised syllabus ER1991 prescribed by Pharmacy Council of India.

This book is small and humble effort has been put in for compiling necessary information on the subject. An attempt has been made to demystify and simplify the basic concepts for the students of pharmacy and to enable them get an evergreen success in MSBTE examinations.

The salient features of the present book are:

- Lucid and easy language
- To the point answers
- Remembering facts in the simplest way
- Infusing confidence in the reader to appear in the Board Examinations.

Hence the series is named

CBS Confident Pharmacy Series

I am confident that this book will be useful to both the students and the teachers of Diploma in Pharmacy as well as the candidates desiring to succeed in competitive examinations for better job opportunities in pharmacy profession such as hospital pharmacists in PHCs, civil hospitals, etc.

Raje Vijay N

Acknowledgements

I express my heartfelt thanks to Prof Madan Jagtap, Chairman, Gourishankar Education Society, Satara Maharashtra, for consistent encouragement and inspiration for writing this book.

I wish to acknowledge the prompt and efficient help given by Prof Milind Jagtap, Mr Jaywant Salunkhe, Mr Appa Rajage, Mr Nitin Mudalgikar, and Mr Shrirang Katekar of Gourishankar Education Society, Satara.

I am also thankful to Shri Satish Kumar Jain, Chairman and Managing Director, and Shri RN Mandal, General Manager, Pune Branch, CBS Publishers & Distributors Pvt Ltd, for their sustained efforts and keen interest in the publication of this book.

I wish all my beloved students to have a great success in the Board Examinations.

Raje Vijay N

Syllabus

(As per ER 1991)

Hospital and Clinical Pharmacy

Part I: Hospital Pharmacy

1. Hospitals—Definition, function, classifications based on various criteria, organisation, management and helath delivery system in India.
2. Hospital pharmacy
   (a) Definition
   (b) Functions and objectives of hospital pharmaceutical services
   (c) Location, layout, flow chart of materials and men
   (d) Personnel and facilities requirements including equipment based on individual and basic needs.
   (e) Requirements and abilities required for hospital pharmacists.
3. Drug Distribution system in hospitals
   (a) Out-patient services
   (b) In-patient services: (i) Types of services (ii) detailed discussion of unit dose system, Floor ward stock system, Satellite pharmacy services, Central sterile services, Bed side pharmacy.
4. Manufacturing
   (a) Economical considerations, estimation of demand
   (b) Sterile manufacture, large and small volume parenterals, facilities, requirements, layout, production planning, man-power requirements.
   (c) Non-sterile manufacture—Liquid orals, externals, bulk concentrates.
   (d) Procurement of stores and testing of raw materials.
5. Nomenclature and uses of surgical instruments and hospital equipment and health accessories.
6. PTC (Pharmacy Therapeutic Committee), Hospital Formulary System and their organisation, functioning, composition.
7. Drug information service and drug information bulletin.

Surgical dressing like cotton, gauze, bandages and adhesive tapes including their pharmacopoeial test for quality. Other hospital supply, e.g. IV sets, BG sets, Ryals tubes, Catheters, Syringes.

Application of computers in maintenance of records, inventory control, medication monitoring, drug information and data storage and retrieval in hospital and retail pharmacy establishments.

Part II: Clinical Pharmacy

1. Introduction to clinical pharmacy practice—Definition, scope.
2. Modern dispensing aspects—Pharmacists and patient counselling and advice for the use of common drugs, medication history.
3. Common daily terminology used in the practice of medicine.
4. Disease, manifestations and pathophysiology including salient symptoms to understand the diseases like tuberculosis, hepatitis, rheumatoid arthritis, cardiovascular diseases, epilepsy, diabetes, peptic ulcer, hypertension.
5. Physiological parameters with their significance.
6. Drugs interactions
   (a) Definition and introduction
   (b) Mechanism of drug interaction
   (c) Drug-drug interaction with reference to analgesics, diuretics, cardiovascular drugs. Gastrointrestinal agent, vitamins and hypoglycemic agents.
   (d) Drug-food interaction.
7. Adverse drug reactions
   (a) Definition and significance
   (b) Drug-induced diseases and teratogenicity
8. Drugs in clinical toxicity—Introduction, general treatment of poisoning, systematic antidotes. Treatment insecticide poisoning heavy metal poison, narcotic drugs, barbiturate, organophosphorus poisons.
9. Drug dependences, drug abuse, addicive drugs and their treatment complications.
10. Bio-availability of drugs, including factors affecting it.

Contents

Part I

Hospital Pharmacy

1

Hospital

1 **Define hospital. State the functions of modern hospital. (S. 96, 97, 98, 00,01, 02, 04; W. 97, 00, 01, 02, 03, 04, 06)**

☞ Hospital

According to WHO, "hospital is an organization of governing body which makes the use of complicated but specialized scientific equipments and functioning through a team of trained staff".

Hospital is an organization which provides a special facility and working for care of patient through the trained persons.

Functions of Modern Hospital

1. To take a care of sick and injured patients.
2. Restoring and keeping up good health of community.
3. To promote good services to patient for getting relief from diseases and pains.
4. To lower the incidences of diseases through early detection and treatment.
5. To make trained and skilled physicians and nurses.
6. To maintain and distribute hospital formulary.
7. To promote research in medical, pharmaceutical and other related fields.
8. To take care of patient by using advanced knowledge and instruments.
9. To rise general standard of medicine for increasing quality of patient care.

10. To contribute in prevention of spreading of disease in the community.
11. To run the programmes like public education and vaccination.
12. It serves as a link between community and official health agencies to improve community health.
13. The bigger hospitals co-operate with smaller hospitals. Thus, hospital performs co-operative work.
14. Primary function is to take care of inpatients and outpatients.

2 Give the classification of hospital. (S. 96, 97, 01, 02, 03, 04, 05, 07, 09; W. 96, 00, 02, 05)

☞ Hospital

A. On Clinical Basis

1. Types of disease

(i) TB hospitals.
(ii) Mental hospitals.
(iii) Leprosy hospitals.
(iv) Cancer hospitals.

2. Types of patient

(i) Gynaecological hospitals.
(ii) Maternity hospitals.
(iii) Pediatric hospitals.

3. Types of medicine

(i) Allopathic hospitals.
(ii) Ayurvedic hospitals.
(iii) Homeopathic hospitals.
(iv) Unani hospitals.
(v) Nature-cure centers
(vi) Physiotherapy centers.

4. Types of organ

(i) ENT hospitals.
(ii) Eye hospitals.
(iii) Orthopaedic hospitals.
(iv) Kidney hospitals.

B. On Non-Clinical Basis

1. On the basis of ownership (S. 96, 06, 08; W. 04, 06)

(a) *Govt:*

(i) Central government Railway and defence hospitals.

(ii) State government: Civil hospitals.
(iii) Local government: Municipality hospitals.

(b) *Non-Government*:

(i) Run by trust.
(ii) Run by limited company.
(iii) Run by religious body.
(iv) Other private hospitals/nursing homes.

2. On the basis of size (bed capacity) (W. 96)

(i) Large hospitals: > 1000 beds, e.g. KEM Hospital (1600 beds).
(ii) Medium hospitals: 500 to 1000 beds, e.g. Bombay Hospital (700 beds).
(iii) Small hospitals: 100 to 500 beds, e.g. Hinduja Hospital (175 beds).
(iv) Very small hospitals: Less than 100 beds, e.g. PMD Hospital (75 beds).

3. On the basis of cost

(i) Elite hospitals: Hospitalisation rates vary between Rs 500–1200 per day.
(Like five-star hotels with facilities like TV, telephone, fridge, etc.) e.g. Jaslok and Hinduja Hospital.
(ii) Low budget hospitals: Civil hospitals, corporation hospitals.

C. Miscellaneous Hospitals

1. Accredited hospitals

These hospitals provide facilities which are decided by council about the health care. In United States such hospitals are present.

2. Others

(i) Teaching hospitals.
(ii) General hospitals, e.g. Civil Hospital.
(iii) Hospitals for non-profit purpose, e.g. Ramakrishna Mission Hospital, Kolkata.
(iv) Hospitals for profit purpose.

3 Write a note on 'organization of hospital'. (S. 96, 01, 03; W. 00, 02)

☞• The hospital is run by the governing body or by the board of trustee or by society, trust or association.

- The governing body members are having experience, knowledge and qualification from several fields.
- The governing body/board of trustee is legally responsible for the specific activities run by the trust.
- For smooth functioning of hospital, governing body appoints the qualified and experienced person as the head of particular institution of hospital.
- Head of the hospital is called hospital administrator/director/dean of the hospital. He is the experienced and qualified person from clinical field. Mainly he/she should be having master degree from medical field and minimum 6 to 10 years experience.
- Hospital administrator is selected or appointed by governing body and is coopted by governing body as its member.
- The heads of all departments are the assistants of administrator.
- The department heads are having minimum master degree from their fields and they are assisted by other staff.
- The departments are classified as clinical and non-clinical departments.
- *Clinical departments:* Gynaecological department, paediatric department, ophthalmic department, surgery department. *Non-clinical departments*: Pharmacy department, nursing department, laundry department, radiology department, maintenance department, etc.
- The staff pattern of each department is different and dependant on the type of services given by the department. The heads of departments are assisted by assistant heads and staff of that department.
- For radiology department, head is assisted by assistant head and other two or three technicians.
- For nursing department, the staff pattern is large. The head of nursing department is assisted by concerned assistant heads and nurses. Generally, one nurse should be made available for maximum 3 patients only. Therefore, on the basis of bed capacity of depatment, staff pattern of nursing department, pharmacy department is to be decided.
- For taking decision in emergency conditions and other complicated conditions the committees were prepared such as:
  - (i) Temporary committees, e.g. building construction committee, joint conference committee.

(ii) Permanent committees, e.g. executive committee, PTC, finance committee.

- Thus, the organisation of hospital is dependant on type of services offered by hospital, bed capacity of hospital.

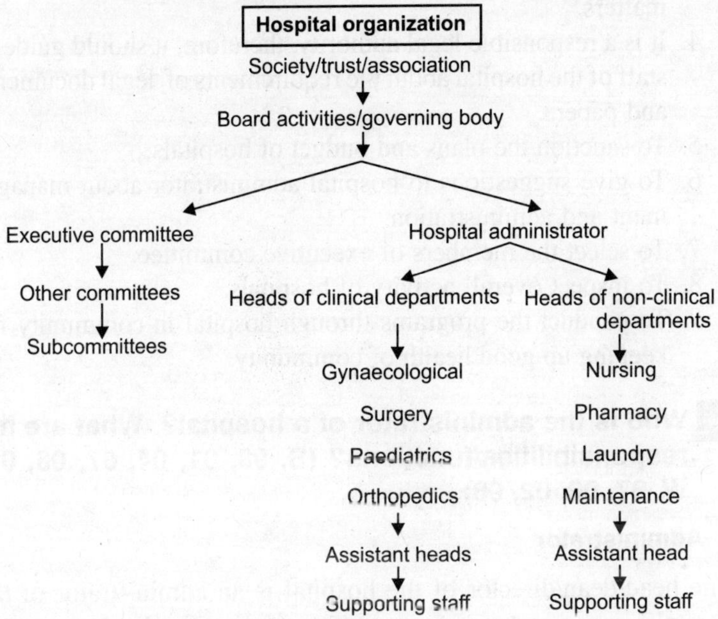

4 Write the constitution and functions of governing body of the hospital.

- Governing body is organization having legal authority about the functioning of hospital.
- It is prepared by trust/association/society.
- It is prepared to control over the functioning of hospital.

Constitution

- It is generally constituted by persons from medical, pharmacy, nursing and other fields.
- The governing body coopts some persons which are well known in specific fields, e.g. social workers and advocates.
- The members of this committee should have an interest in social and legal functioning of the hospital. These members should indirectly increase the status of hospital in community.

Functions of Governing Body

1. To appoint hospital administrator.
2. To establish objectives of hospitals.
3. To answer about queries asked by the court regarding court matters.
4. It is a responsible legal authority, therefore, it should guide to staff of the hospital about the requirements of legal documents and papers.
5. To sanction the plans and budget of hospitals.
6. To give suggestions to hospital administrator about management and administration.
7. To select the members of executive committee.
8. To inspect overall activity of hospitals.
9. To conduct the programs through hospital in community for keeping up good health of community.

5 Who is the administrator of a hospital? What are his responsibilities/functions? (S. 98, 01, 04, 07, 08, 09; W. 97, 00, 02, 08)

☞ Administrator

"The head/dean/director of the hospital is an administrator of the hospital."

- He is a member of governing body.
- He is the head of PTC.
- He is the secretary of joint and executive committees.
- He is a qualified and experienced person from medical field.
- He is having minimum master degree in medical field and 6 to 10 years experience.

Functions/Responsibility/Role of Hospital Administrator

1. To implement the policies of the governing body.
2. To decide the subcommittees, their members and functions.
3. To decide scientific programmes for the development of knowledge of staff.
4. To manage routine activities by considering main purpose of patient care.
5. To appoint heads of department by taking consideration of governing body.

6. To attend seminars, meetings arranged by other hospitals.
7. To arrange the programmes for keeping good health of the community and to increase the status of hospital.
8. To decide the programmes for training of physicians, nurses and volunteers and control over such programmes and activities.
9. To communicate with hospital staff and to discuss about problems of staff.
10. To attend the meetings of the governing body and to discuss about budget of hospital, finance and other problems of hospital.
11. To take sanctions or approvals of governing body for hospital budget.
12. To check the documents and activities done in hospitals.
13. He should plan for the expansion of a hospital.
14. He should coordinates the work of various section heads of the hospital.
15. He has to provide facilities, equipment and assistancc to clinical department.

6 What are different types of services provided by hospital? (W. 00, 02)

☞ The services provided by hospital are divided into two categories:

Clinical services	Non-clinical services (supportive services)
(i) General surgery and orthopaedic (ii) Gynaecologic and obstetrics (iii) ENT (iv) Ophthalmologic (v) Anaesthesia (vi) Psychiatric and nervous diseases (vii) Tuberculosis (viii) Communical diseases (ix) Paediatric (x) Medical services (staff pattern)	(i) Nursing services (ii) Dietary services (iii) Pharmacy (iv) Housekeeping services (v) Pathological services (vi) Blood bank (vii) Anaesthesia service (viii) Account keeping service

1. Clinical Services

Clinical services are completely governed by medically trained and qualified doctors who diagnose and treat the patient.

(i) **General surgery:** Surgical services are offered by surgical department and useful for better care and easy to overcome symptoms of diseases. These services are provided by professionally trained and experience doctors. They are assisted by a number of physicians, nurses and compounders.

(ii) **Medical services (staff pattern)**: The staff pattern is dependent on type of patient. The staff is classified as:

(a) ***Honorary staff*:** It consists of physicians who are active in hospital during their working years and having interest to work after retirement and having their outstanding performance and experience.

(b) ***Consulting staff*:** These are specialized from specific faculty and available for specified time only.

(c) ***Active staff*:** These are active and full time employees of the hospital. These are having involvement to increase the standard of hospitals.

(d) ***Associated medical staff*:** These are junior and less experienced physicians.

(e) ***Residential medical staff*:** These are the group of physicians who are employees of hospital and living in campus of hospitals.

(f) ***Courtesy medical staff*:** It is the group of physicians who had decided to attend the private patient but refuse the membership of hospital.

2. Non-clinical Services (Supportive Services)

(a) **Nursing services:** This service provides the total health care to patient. It is a therapeutic and preventive service. The emotional support to the patient is also provided by this department. The in-charge of this department is a coordinator between medical and nursing staff. The head of this department should perform following functions:

(i) Select the procedure and policies of nursing.
(ii) To keep the nursing records.
(iii) To prepare required budget.
(iv) To provide nursing supplies to nurses.
(v) To discuss about nursing problems with the director of hospital.
(vi) To adjust departmental duties of nurses.

(vii) To take part in seminars for getting the recent knowledge.
(viii) To train the nursing staff.

(b) **Dietary services:** It is a therapeutic service offered by the hospital. The food is offered on scientific basis to each inpatient and suggestions are given about the diet by the food manager. The head of this department is called dietitian.

The duties of head of this department are:

(i) To perform the plan for the type of diet for the patient by considering his food allergies and dietary histories.
(ii) Selection and purchasing of food materials.
(iii) Maintenance of record about purchasing and utilization of food material.
(iv) To act as authority for preparation and distribution of diet to each patient.
(v) To train and to supervise over the staff of the department.
(vi) To follow the specific precautions about the storage of food material.
(vii) To help in research studies.

The head of this department should have master degree and at least 2 years experience the staff of this department should be at least 12% of the total hospital staff. The prepared food is transferred to nursing department for distribution.

(c) **Pharmacy services:** This department is governed by the head of department of pharmacology. It stores and dispenses medications and other supplies to inpatients as well as to outpatients.

(d) **Housekeeping services:** It provides cleaned and clear hospital and bed making services. The head of this department is called housekeeper. Housekeeper is well known and educated person. He is having the knowledge of cleansing agents, detergents, disinfectants, soaps, etc.

His duties are:

(i) To coordinate with other departmental staff.
(ii) To keep records about the utilization of cleansing agents, beds, pillow covers, bed sheets, etc.
(iii) To adjust the duties of departmental staff.
(iv) To train the unskilled workers.

(e) **Pathological services:** Head of this department is a medical person with special training in pathology. It provides services such as checking of blood, urine, stool samples of the patients.

(f) **Blood bank:** Most of the hospitals operate blood bank facilities under department of pathology.

(g) **Anaesthesia services:** Head of this department is a specially qualified and trained medical person also known as anaesthetist. They provide anaesthesia services required during surgery.

(h) **Account keeping services:** This department controls over intake and the utilization of money. This department manages purchasing medicines, instruments and other hospital supply and expenses over maintenance of hospital, payments of employees, etc.

7 Write in general management and organisation of "health delivery system in India". (S. 06; W. 04, 05, 06, 08).

☞ Health delivery system in India is managed by government agencies and private agencies.

In central or state government run hospitals, the controlling is under health ministry headed by central or state health minister.

At district level, there is a chief medical officer (CMO), assistant district medical officer (AMO), primary health centre (PHC), in-charge medical officer.

At the hospital level itself, a dean or director or medical officer is the controlling authority.

Health Delivery System in India

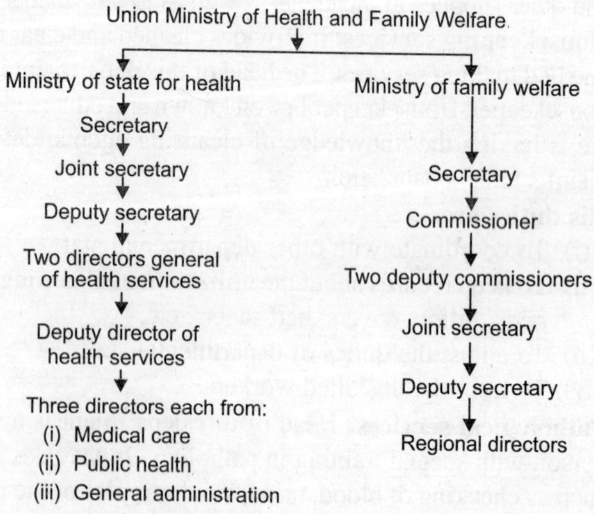

8 Give the organization of "health delivery system at state level". (W. 04)

☞ Health minister

↓

Deputy minister

↓

Health secretary-incharge

↓

Deputy secretary

↓

Director of health services

↓

Deputy director of health services

↓

Eight assistant directors of health services

↓

(1) Medical education
(2) Nursing
(3) Mother/child health
(4) Family welfare
(5) Nutrition
(6) School health
(7) Primary health centres
(8) Health education.

Health delivery system at state level

2

Hospital Pharmacy

1 Define hospital pharmacy. Give objectives and functions of hospital pharmacy. (S. 96, 97, 98, 99, 01, 02, 05, 06, 07, 09; W. 96, 98, 99, 00, 04, 05, 06, 08)

☞ Hospital Pharmacy

"It is the department which receives medicines and other supplies, stores them and dispenses to the inpatients and outpatients and may have manufacturing extension."

Objectives

1. To provide the right medicine to right patient at right time, in right quantity with minimum cost.
2. To plan, organize and implement the policies of pharmacy.
3. To implement the decision of PTC.
4. To participate in research work.
5. To act as profit centre of the hospital.
6. To act as a counselling centre to the patient.
7. To act as an information centre about drugs.
8. To manufacture large volume parenterals or suitable dosage forms.

Functions

1. To participate in patient care system by dispensing medicine and monitoring the patient.
2. Dispensing of narcotics, medicines and pharmaceutical preperations.

3. Dispensing of radiopharmaceuticals and alcohol-containing drugs.
4. Dispensing of surgical dressing and related products.
5. Packaging of medicines, drugs and labelling of containers.
6. It acts as a profit centre of the hospital.
7. Checking and maintaining of records of drugs about utilization, distribution, etc.
8. Maintenance of inventory control, purchasing methods, book keeping and record keeping.
9. To check sources of drugs and medicines.
10. To check the received materials for their standards.
11. To implement decision of PTC and maintain the distribution system of drugs.
12. To furnish the information about drugs to the patients and clarify queries asked by patients and thus it acts as information and counselling centre.
13. Manufacturing of sterile and nonsterile products and checking of prepared products.
14. To take part in research study and to cooperate with other departments.
15. To take part in various programmes arranged by hospital for better community health.

2 Give the location and layout of hospital pharmacy department. (S. 03; W. 96, 99, 01)

☞ Location

- Hospital pharmacy department should be located at ground floor or at first floor of the hospital.
- It should be away from inpatient department.
- It should be near to outpatient department, hospital library, drug information centre and should be attached to the manufacturing unit of hospital pharmacy.
- The space for hospital pharmacy department should be minimum 250 sq. feet as per schedule N.
- Depending upon the bed capacity of the hospital the area for hospital pharmacy department is as follows:
  - (i) For 100 bed hospital, 10 sq. feet per bed.
  - (ii) For 200 bed hospital 6 to 8 sq. feet per bed.

- According to bed capacity of hospital, type of work and workload norms, the requirement of pharmacist is fulfilled.
- At least 3 pharmacists should be appointed for any small hospital.
- According to bed capacity the number of pharmacists required are:

Up to 50 beds	—	3 pharmacists
Up to 100 beds	—	5 pharmacists
Up to 200 beds	—	8 pharmacists
Up to 300 beds	—	10 pharmacists
Up to 500 beds	—	15 pharmacists.

- Generally, outpatient attendance and bed strength ratio is 3:1. One pharmacist can be recommended for maximum 10 patients.

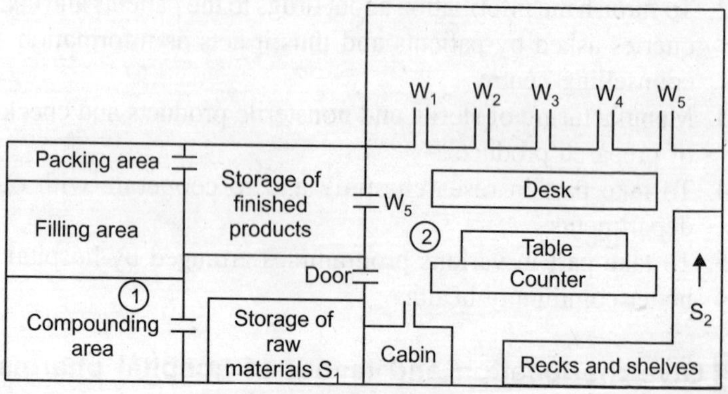

Layout of hospital pharmacy department

Section 1.= Manufacturing department
2.= Hospital pharmacy
W_1 and W_2 = Dispensing to outpatients
W_3 = For dispensing to inpatients
W_4 = Dispensing to emergency patients
W_5 = For getting medicines to dispensing from manufacturing section
S_1 = Storage of raw materials
S_2 = Storage of drugs and medicines

- Due to location of hospital pharmacy at ground floor, easy dispensing to the outpatient and to other departments is possible.
- Hospital pharmacy should have adequate space separately for cold storage, storage of narcotic drugs, radiopharmaceuticals, manufacturing section, for outpatient dispensing, for labelling,

packing weighing and compounding, for central sterile supply, for officer in-charge of hospital pharmacy and for hospital library.

- The hospital pharmacy department should have pleasant look and enough space and furniture.
- The educative posters, informative hanging charts should be adjusted on walls, to fill up the waiting time.
- The light literatures, newspapers, educative magazines should be provided in waiting rooms.
- The floors and walls should be clean.
- The floor should be acid-resistant and wall should be painted by light colour and should have smooth surface.
- If manufacturing section is started in hospital, it should be attached to main pharmacy department.
- In large hospitals separate pharmacy substations are located at each floor. Such substations are in vertical manner therefore, stair way connection can be adjusted.

3 Give the flow chart of materials.

☞ • Hospital pharmacy receives its supply of materials either from outside manufacturing units or manufacturing units present inside the hospitals.

Flow chart of materials

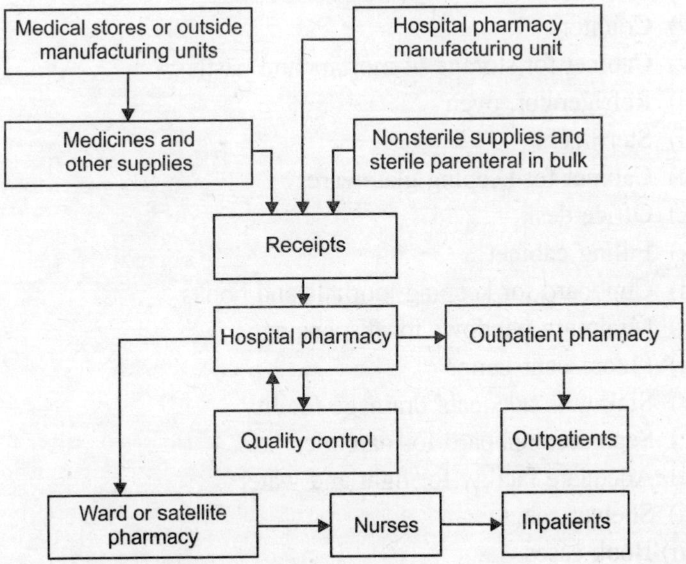

- These supplies are stored and dispensed according to the need to the inpatients or outpatients ultimately.
- It keeps quality control over the receipts.
- For inpatients the supplies are provided through nurses through the ward pharmacies.
- Outpatients medications are supplied through the outpatient pharmacy.

4 What are the requirements of space and equipment for smooth working of hospital pharmacy? (S. 98; W. 97)

☞ The type of hospital, bed capacity of hospital decide the space for pharmacy department. As per schedule N the space for pharmacy department should be minimum 250 sq. feet.

The separate area should be provided to dispensing and distribution, for drug store, for subdepartments of pharmacy. If manufacturing section is also opened in hospital, separate equipments and space should be provided to that section as per the norms.

Facilities and Equipment Required for Dispensing and Distribution

(i) Prescription cabinet
(ii) Storage cabinet
(iii) Working table
(iv) Counters
(v) Cabinet for storage of mortars and pastles
(vi) Refrigerator, oven
(vii) Sterilizers
(viii) Cabinet for keeping glasswares
(ix) Office desk
(x) Filling cabinet
(xi) Cupboard for keeping journals and books
(xii) Minimum windows for dispensing
(xiii) Fluorescent lamps
(xiv) Sink with adequate drainage facility
(xv) Separate cupboard for narcotics
(xvi) Adequate facility for light and water
(xvii) Shelves rakes
(xviii) Book cases

(xix) Lockers
(xx) Notice boards.

For Manufacturing Section

(i) Containers for manufacturing
(ii) Containers and closures
(iii) Packaging material
(iv) Balances for weighing
(v) Machineries required for manufacturing and packing
(vi) Water distillation stills.

For Sterile Products/Section

(i) UV lamps
(ii) Laminar flow
(iii) Bacteria-proof filters
(iv) Aseptic cabinet, etc.

Requirement of Pharmacists/Personnel

The pharmacist should be engaged with maximum 10 patients. The number of pharmacists required is:

Up to 50 beds	:	3 Pharmacists
Up to 100 beds	:	5 Pharmacists
Up to 200 beds	:	8 Pharmacists
Up to 500 beds	:	15 Pharmacists

Separate pharmacist for the dispensing, distribution, drug store, manufacturing section, clinical pharmacy, drug information centre, quality control should be available.

5 Describe the qualification requirements and abilities required for hospital pharmacists (head of hospital pharmacy). (S. 00, 03, 05; W. 96, 98, 99, 00, 03, 05, 06, 08)

☞ The head of hospital pharmacy department should be at least M Pharm in pharmacology. Clinical pharmacist should have a degree such as master in clinical pharmacy. Quality control incharge should be M Pharma (analytical chemistry) and assistants should be B Pharm or D Pharm. The head of hospital pharmacy should have following abilities:

(i) Administrative ability.
(ii) Technical ability.

(iii) Academic ability.
(iv) Ability to develop manufacturing section.
(v) Ability to control.

Administrative Ability

- He should have an ability to plan, organize, direct and to control over various activities and functions of hospital pharmacy department.
- He should have an ability to select the staff for pharmacy department and to train and guide them.
- He should prepare proper work schedule, purchasing, budget and should develop better pricing system for costing of prescription.
- He should have an ability to interact properly with other departments.
- He should motivate his staff for achieving greater heights in functioning of pharmacy.
- He should have an ability to make pharmacy department as economical viable unit.
- He should have information about the government rules and regulations for proper record-keeping related with drug distribution, purchasing, utilization, etc.

Technical Ability

- He should have adequate knowledge about the storage of drugs, drug interactions, precautions, dose of drugs.
- He should develop proper drug distribution system, proper way of dispensing and good pricing system of medicines.
- He should know pharmacokinetic, pharmacodynamic, pharmacological and pharmacotherapeutic aspects of drugs.
- He should clarify the queries asked by the assistants or physicians.

Academic Ability

- He is the head of department therefore, he is also responsible for better manufacturing, dispensing procedures.
- He should have ability to develop suitable training programmes for pharmacist.
- He should have an ability to guide pharmacy staff to conduct active research useful for development of product, dispensing and pricing system.

- He should motivate his staff for medical and pharmaceutical research.
- He should provide research and training material to the staff.
- He should take part in seminars and programmes arranged by the hospital.
- He should know about research methodology.
- He should provide motivation to the staff in taking patient care and to perform better functioning of the departments.
- He should have an ability to train the staff of the department.

Ability to Develop Manufacturing Section

- He should have knowledge about the pharmaceutics.
- He should have an ability to prepare the estimate for starting manufacturing section.
- He should know the standards required for manufacturing of particular dosage forms.
- He should know about the instruments and machinery, apparatus required for the manufacturing of dosage forms.
- He should have an ability to attract a suitable person as the head of manufacturing section.

Ability to Control

- He should have control over the inventory of drugs and over the money expenditure.
- He should have an ability to develop suitable procedure for purchasing of drugs, costing of prescription, etc.
- He should have an ability to control over the staff of his department.
- He should be able to inspect any subpharmacy department at any time.
- He should maintain smooth functioning of pharmacy department.

6 Write in brief about organization of hospital pharmacy department.

☞ The organization pattern of hospital pharmacy department depends upon the duties and functions carried out by the hospital pharmacy department.

Separate pharmacist should be engaged as the head of the department.

In large hospitals the separate in-charge for each department appointed.

- The head of hospital pharmacy department should be M Pharm in pharmacology with adequate abilities like administrative ability, technical ability, etc.

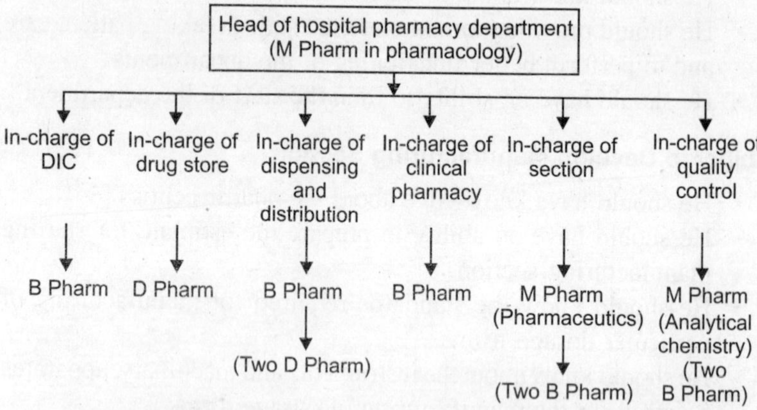

- The head of hospital pharmacy department is assited by heads of dispensing and distribution and also of DIC, drug store, clinical pharmacy, quality control and manufacturing unit.
- The head of drug store should be D Pharm and that of manufacturing section, M Pharm in pharmaceutics. The heads from other subdepartments should be at least B Pharm.
- Only quality control department should have a head from analytical chemistry and at least a master degree in pharmacy (M Pharm).
- In-charge of manufacturing section is assisted by two bachelor in pharmacy, in-charge of quality control section is assisted by two B Pharms.
- In-charge of dispensing and distribution is assisted by two D Pharms.
- As per workload the staff pattern may be changed.
- In manufacturing section helpers and other assistants are more as compared to sections such as DIC, etc.
- The quality control department requires assistants for performing analysis and checking of every incoming material and finished products.

3

Drug Distribution System in Hospitals

1 Define outpatient. Explain/give types of outpatients (classify). (S. 96, 97, 02, 06, 09; W. 98, 02, 08)

☞ Outpatient

"The patient which is not admitted in hospital but receiving general or specific treatment is called outpatient."

Classification of Outpatient

(i) **General outpatient:** The outpatients which are not receiving emergency or specific treatment are called general outpatients, e.g. diabetic patient, hypertension patient.

(ii) **Emergency outpatient:** The outpatients if receiving emergency treatment or an accident care are called emergency outpatients.

(iii) **Referred outpatients:** If outpatients are receiving specific treatment then those are called reffered outpatients, e.g. patients suffering from eye, ear, nose, teeth disorders.

(iv) **Ambulatory patient:** "An ambulatory patient is 'able to walk' and since outpatients receive primary health care and walk off, they are wrongly called ambulatory patients."

Majority of outpatients are ambulatory patients.

2 Give the location and layout of outpatient dispensing.

☞ Location

- There should be separate independent outpatient pharmacy.

- If inpatient and outpatient services are combined, separate windows should be provided for dispensing.
- The outpatients dispensing is done from the same pharmacy where stock preparations are made.
- There should be two prescription windows, one for men and other for women.
- The pharmacy receives its supplies from medical stores for at least a week and emergency supplies at any time.
- In some hospitals, outpatient department and pharmacy are separated geographically.
- In such situation, it is necessary to have an autonomous outpatient pharmacy.
- Combined services of inpatients–outpatients are better to control for chief pharmacist.
- The outpatient department should be located in such a way that, it should not cause disturbance to the inpatients.

Layout of OPD

- Layout of OPD creates an image of the hospital.
- It shows the quality of service provided by hospital.
- In the layout there should be adequate number of windows for receiving and filling up prescriptions.
- Layout should be such that, patient traffic can be easily controlled.
- Waiting time of outpatients should be reduced.
- Waiting rooms should be pleasantly furnished with sufficient reading material and educative posters hanged on the walls form an integral part of the OPD.
- To avoid overcrowding, more windows and manpower should be provided.

3 Enlist different methods of drug distribution system to inpatients in hospitals. (S. 97, 01; W. 98, 02, 03)

☞ 1. Individual prescription order system.
2. Floor stock/ward stock system
   (i) Charged floor stock system.
   (ii) Non-charged floor stock system.
3. Combined individual prescription order system and floor stock system.

4. Unit dose dispensing system (UDDS)
   (i) Centralized unit dose dispensing system (CUDDS)
   (ii) Decentralized unit dose dispensing system (DCUDDS)
5. Satellite pharmacy
6. Bedside pharmacy.

4 Describe individual prescription order system/individual prescription medication for patient as distribution system in hospitals.

☞ Individual Prescription Order System

- Small and private hospitals adapt this system.
- According to this system prescription is received by pharmacist and medicines are dispensed for inpatients.
- The collection of prescription is also done by pharmacist.
- Here the drugs are dispensed and labeled for each individual patient.
- Here medications are kept in nursing unit medication cabinet under the custody of nurse in-charge.
- Nurse is responsible for administering correct medications to each patient in ward.
- The nurses are advised by the pharmacist about proper storage, labeling and accounting of drugs and unwanted effect produced by drug, etc.
- For faster dispensing, commonly used drugs can be prepackaged.

Advantages

(i) Review of prescription is possible by the pharmacist.
(ii) Pharmacist can counsel the patient.
(iii) Control over inventory is easy.
(iv) Purchasing cost, maintenance cost, space required are less in comparison with other systems.
(v) Maintenance of record is easy and paper work is minimized.
(vi) Patient should pay for the medicines which are consumed by him.
(vii) Adjustment of cost of prescription is possible by considering economical condition of the patient.

Disadvantages

(i) Emergency medicines are not quickly supplied.
(ii) Delay in receiving medicines.

(iii) Waiting period for the patient is increased.
(iv) Prepackaging requires more man power.

Application

Useful in small and private hospitals.

5 Write a note on floor stock/ward stock system. (S. 96, 01, 02, 06; W. 96, 01, 02, 03, 04)

☞ Floor Stock System

"It is the system where drugs are stored at each floor or near to the ward at nursing stations."

Method

1. At the end of the day pharmacist should collect the requisition and empty containers from the various nursing units.
2. These containers are filled and on next morning the medicines are given to nursing station.
3. Generally at night, while leaving the duty, pharmacist should collect the requisition and empty containers and on next morning the next pharmacist supplies medicines and containers to the nursing unit.
4. This system is followed for 2 to 3 times per week or according to requirement.

Types of Floor Stock System

PTC decides types of floor stock medicines as:

(a) **Charged floor stock:** If charged floor stock medicines are given to the patient, cost of those medicines is directly added to the patient's account, e.g. includes cost medicines such as penicillin, streptomycin, quinidine, diuretics, tranquillizers, etc.
- PTC decides charged floor stock drugs and its requirement.
- The selected list of charged floor stock is constantly being reviewed by the PTC for necessary revision.

(b) **Non-charged floor stock:** These medications are stocked on nursing stations at all times, but they are not directly charged to an account of patient. The cost of such medicines is adjusted in the room rent, e.g. saline solutions, dextrose solutions are non-charged drugs.

Selection of Non-charged Floor Stock System

Criteria

(i) Cost of the product.
(ii) Frequency of use.
(iii) Quantity of use.
(iv) Effect on hospital budget.
(v) Type of product.

Advantages of Floor Stock System

(i) Waiting period is less. Medicines can be received immediately.
(ii) Emergency medicines are easily available for quick distribution.
(iii) Number of pharmacists required for dispensing are reduced.
(iv) It avoids exercise of patient's relatives to bring the medications.

Disadvantages of Floor Stock System

(i) Review of prescription by pharmacist is not possible.
(ii) Inventory is increased therefore, budget of hospital is increased.
(iii) Counseling of patient by pharmacist is not possible.
(iv) Paper work is increased.
(v) More space is required at nursing station for stocking medicines.
(vi) Maintenance cost and wastage of medicines is increased.
(vii) Medication errors are not minimized.
(viii) It increases work load of nurses.

Applications

(i) Useful in large hospitals.
(ii) Helps to check the efficacy of nursing unit.
(iii) It provides emergency supply of medicines to the patient.

6 Write a note on 'unit dose dispensing system' (UDDS). (S. 96, 97, 99, 01, 02, 03, 04, 05, 07, 09; W. 97, 98, 02, 03, 06, 08)

☞ Definition

It is the system which consists of dispensing unit doses to the patients containing a predetermined amount of drug.

- These unit doses are either stored or distributed from main pharmacy department only.

- The solid ingredients are repacked and liquids are remeasured.
- Unit doses are prepared as per the requirement.
- It is useful to inpatients and also to outpatients.

Types of Unit Dose Dispensing System

(a) **Centralized unit dose dispensing system (CUDDS):** If the unit doses are dispensed from pharmacy department, it is called centralized unit dose dispensing system.

(b) **Decentralized unit dose dispensing system (DCUDDS):** If the unit doses are dispensed from nursing stations, it is called decentralized unit dose dispensing system.

Advantages of Unit Dose Dispensing System

(i) Avoids misuse of medication.
(ii) Review of prescription is possible therefore, medication errors are reduced.
(iii) Time required for dispensing is reduced.
(iv) Patient should pay the cost of medicines which are consumed by him.
(v) Purchasing cost and budget of hospital is decreased.
(vi) Accounting becomes easier.
(vii) Paper work is less at nursing unit as well as at the pharmacy.
(viii) Better financial control.

Disadvantages of Unit Dose Dispensing System

(i) Separate manpower is required for prepackaging.
(ii) Separate containers, closures, machinery and also space is required.
(iii) Unit dispensing should be handled by skilled person and supervised by pharmacist only.

Benefits of UDDS

(i) The patients are charged only for those medications which are consumed by them.
(ii) It reduces the medication error since the pharmacist checks a copy of physician's original order.
(iii) It avoids wastage of drug.
(iv) Less space is required as compared to bulky floor stock.
(v) It allows the nurses more time for direct patient care.

(vi) Patient receives the nursing service 24 hours a day.
(vii) It avoids the duplication of orders and extra paper work.
(viii) It increases more efficient utilization of personnel.

7 What is satellite pharmacy? (S. 97, 98, 99, 01, 04, 05; W. 96, 98, 00, 01, 03)

☞ Definition

The main pharmacy centre is called satellite pharmacy and sub-pharmacy centers are located at each floor and working as substations for satellite.

Satellite pharmacy service is developed with an advanced view of clinical pharmacy programs. These subpharmacies are located on wards. They receive their supply from main pharmacy and distribute them to the patients on current basis.

These pharmacies are managed by clinical pharmacist who is available in his professional capacity for patient counseling.

Advantages

(i) Review of prescription is possible by pharmacist.
(ii) Waiting period is decreased.
(iii) Emergency medicines are quickly available for administration.
(iv) Drug therapy can be monitored by pharmacist.
(v) Pharmacist may counsel the patient.

Disadvantages

(i) Inventory is increased therefore, budget is increased.
(ii) Paper work, maintenance cost are increased.
(iii) Separate space is required for keeping the stock.
(iv) Number of pharmacists required for dispensing are more.

8 Explain in detail bedside pharmacy. (S. 96, 97, 98, 99, 01, 02, 04, 05, 08; W. 96, 98, 00, 03, 05)

☞ Definition

It is the drug distribution system in hospital in which drugs are kept near the bed of the patient so the patient can utilize the drug himself.

- It provides more patient-oriented service.
- An active participation of pharmacist in day to day management of patients at ward level is expected in this system.

- A bedside pharmacist offers advice regarding the action and uses of frequently used drugs to the medical or nursing staff.
- He also gives his own expert evaluation of the prescribed drugs.
- During his ward visit, he can take the feedback from the patient.
- He takes upon the additional responsibility of drug usage and drug information for which he is trained.
- He directs his efforts to safe and efficient use of drugs.
- He corrects the deficiencies in the use of drugs both by patient and prescribers.
- He monitors the drug use by conducting the pharmacokinetic studies.
- A bedside pharmacy is essentially a drug therapy advisor.

Advantages of Bedside Pharmacy

(i) Professional skill of pharmacist is utilized.
(ii) Review of prescription, counselling to patient is possible.
(iii) Control over drug inventory and utilization is easy and done by pharmacist only.
(iv) Professional skill about the pharmacokinetic studies about the drug interactions, ADR, etc. is used by pharmacist to avoid the medication errors in prescription and simultaneous safe and better use of drug is possible.
(v) Bedside pharmacy system helps to check patient compliance or to improve patient compliance.

Disadvantages

(i) Number of pharmacists required are more in comparison with other systems.
(ii) Chances of over utilization/misuse of drug by patient.

9 Describe in brief central sterile services/central sterile department (CSS/CSD) OR central sterile service room (CSSR). (S. 06, 07, 09; W. 96, 01, 05, 06, 08)

☞ Definition

It is a separate department of hospital providing professional supplies and equipments (sterile and nonsterile) to all specialized departments.

- The items provided by this department include syringes, needles, gloves, bags for urine collection, catheters, cotton pads, blood bottles, etc.

- The equipment distributed by this department are suction pumps, cardiac and other catheters, surgical dressings, trays, monitoring equipment, etc.
- This department is responsible for distribution of medicinal equipments and supply of sterilized materials.
- Central sterile department also takes an active role in developing various gas and cold sterilization techniques.
- The management of central sterile services is under the control of nursing staff, as one of their duties. But a trained pharmacist person is more suitable to maintain sterilization of equipment and preparation of intravenous fluids.

Objectives of Central Sterile Services

(i) To maintain supply of sterile equipments to operation theatre.
(ii) Cleaning and sterilization of all hospital supplies.
(iii) To contribute in educational programs.
(iv) To provide sterile gowns, caps, mask and hand gloves during operations.
(v) To develop cost-effective programme by cost analysis, personal supplies and equipment.

Departments Served by Central Services

(i) Operation theatre.
(ii) Recovery room.
(iii) Intensive surgical care.

Location of Central Sterile Services

- It should be located near the operation theatre.
- It should be located in such a way that most rapid transport of material is possible.
- The department should have capacity to expand itself if the hospital grows in future.
- It should be located near the pharmacy department to have a better administrative control.

Layout of Central Sterile Area (S. 04; W. 96, 05)

[Work-flow pattern of central sterile area.]

The plan of central sterile room is clearly divided into two areas:

1. Nonsterile material area or “dirty area”.
2. Sterile material or “clean area”.

- Through D_2 the material is received by the supply department.
- Received materials are dissembled or kept in the rack.
- Whenever required material is allowed for sterilization, they are kept in the space provided for keeping of sterilized materials.

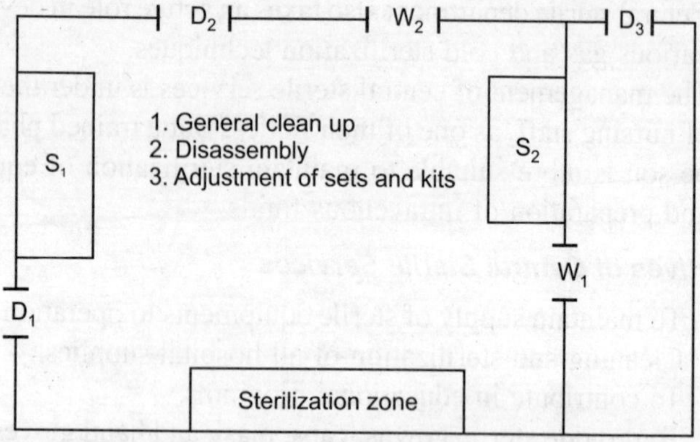

S_1 = Storage of unsterilized materials.
S_2 = Space for storage of sterile materials.
OT = Operation theatre
D_1 and D_2 and D_3 are doors.
W_1 and W_2 are windows.

- The cross flow of sterilized and nonsterilized materials is avoided.
- From W_2 the material is dispensed to departments other than operation theatre and through W_1 sterilized material is supplied to operation theatre.

Functions of Pharmacist in Central Sterile Area

1. Purchasing and receiving hospital supplies and equipment.
2. Storage of hospital supplies and equipment.
3. Dispensing and distribution of hospital supplies to various departments.
4. Maintenance and keeping up the records of purchasing, distribution, etc.
5. Standardization and microbial testing of sterilized products should be done.
6. Interacting with other professionals in health care team.
7. Adjustment of trays for better handling.

10 Give various administrative patterns of central sterile services. (S. 97, 08; W. 02, 08)

☞ 1. **Nursing services:** A nurse should be the head of this department as majority of items are used by nurses for patients.
2. **Pharmacist services:** Though nurse is the head of department, pharmacist also performs important functions, e.g. procurement, storage, distribution of supplies and preparations of various sterile solutions.
3. **Correlation between pharmacist and a nurse:** Some functions of this department like cleaning, packing, distribution of medical supplies and equipment should be placed in charge of a nurse whereas manufacture of sterile solutions should be placed in charge of pharmacists.

11 Write a note on prepackaging. (S. 00; W. 96)

☞ Prepackaging

Prepackaging is an advanced method of distribution and dispensing of fast moving items in the hospitals.

- Prepackaging is also suitable for those items which take a long time for compounding and packaging.
- Prepackaging is adopted only when turnover and demand of the product is more.
- Prepackaging is useful for IPD as well as OPD.
- Prepackaging operation is carried out either by a pharmacist or under his direct supervision.

Advantages of Prepackaging

(i) Increases standard of dispensing in hospitals.
(ii) It is very convenient method.
(iii) It is time-saving.
(iv) It is labour-saving.
(v) Useful in IPD as well as OPD.

Disadvantages of Prepackaging

(i) Once a pack of medicine is given to a patient the remaining quantity in the pack will be wasted.
(ii) Proper storage of drug is necessary.

12 Explain the process of dispensing drugs to outpatients in a typical hospital.

☞ Dispensing of Drugs to Outpatients in Hospital

- Medicines are given to the outpatients from the pharmacy on the prescription given to them by the consultants.
- Free medicine cases directly get medicines but in payment cases they pay the cash at the cash counter and produce the bill along with the prescription to the pharmacy.

Process

1. On entering the hospital, the patient goes to the registration counter, registers his/her name and gets a case paper with the name, sex, age and a number as reference means, identity slip and registration number.
2. On the basis of external symptoms and a few oral questions they are directed to go to a particular department for consultation.
3. Consultant diagnoses the disease and either prescribes the medicines as such or after referring and getting reports from clinical laboratory or radiology department.
4. Next, the patient goes to the cash counter and makes payment.
5. With cash receipt and prescription the patient goes then to pharmacy and gets medicines.
6. The prescription and case paper may be retained here and only registration number and identity slips are given to the patient.
7. The pharmacist sends back the case paper with prescriptions to the registration counter from where the patients get them on their subsequent visit.
8. Schedule 'H' and 'X' drugs dispensing shall need the legal requirements.

4

Manufacturing

STERILE MANUFACTURING

1 **Write in brief about estimation of demand. Explain different methods of estimating demand of hospitals. (S. 97, 02, 04; W. 04)**

☞ Estimation of Demand

- Manufacturing of the sterile and nonsterile pharmaceutical products in a hospital is performed if it is beneficial to the hospital.
- The manufacturing is started under the control of main hospital pharmacy centre.
- Decision about manufacturing of any dosage form is taken by executive committee and governing body.
- Head of hospital pharmacy department prepares estimate of manufacturing of any dosage form. He considers raw materials, packaging materials, manpower, electricity, water requirement, space, machinery, instruments and other requirements and prepares and estimates the budget.
- Manufacturing of dosage form is started if it gives profit to the hospital

Methods of Estimation of Demand

1. **Judgement method:** The judgements and opinions of experts and concerned staff of pharmacy and clinical departments on the past experience about a quantity of product utilized in the hospital are calculated.

2. **Past history analysis:** Past consumption pattern is analyzed. Data are collected yearwise. Further data are evaluated and budget is prepared and demand is estimated.
3. **Causal model method:** It includes both past history and judgement of experts. On the basis of these two studies, exact idea is delivered about the demand of dosage forms, e.g. demand for whole blood is related to admissions in the casualty/ emergency wards, etc.

2 Write a note on "economic considerations" for sterile manufacturing in hospitals. (S. 96, 97, 05, 09; W. 98)

☞ Economic Considerations for Sterile Manufacturing

- Hospital generally starts manufacturing of any dosage form if it is benefited to hospital.
- Economic considerations and budget is prepared by the head of manufacturing section or hospital pharmacy department.
- Total cost is estimated by considering direct and indirect expenses and manufacturing overheads, for total per annum production.
- The budget includes:
  - (i) Cost of raw materials
  - (ii) Manpower (salary)
  - (iii) Direct expenses: Packaging material, instruments
  - (iv) Manufacturing overheads:
    - (a) Rental
    - (b) Repair and maintenance
    - (c) Salaries of employees
    - (d) Water, electricity
    - (e) Sterilization
    - (f) Quality control
    - (g) Cost of laboratory animals and their feed
    - (h) Machines and furniture.
  - (v) Indirect expenses:
    - (a) Office cost
    - (b) Printing
    - (c) Stationary
    - (d) Postage.

Governing body/executive committee analyse and estimate the budget by taking proper economic consideration for manufacturing in hospitals.

3 What is EOQ? Write the formula used to determine EOQ. (S. 97, 00)

☞ EOQ: It is the quantity of item to be purchased where inventory carrying cost and ordering cost are minimum.

It is derived from expected usage cost/unit purchase cost, etc.

$$EOQ = \sqrt{\frac{2US}{ID}}$$

Where,

U = Expected usage
D = Cost/unit
I = Inventory carrying charges
S = Purchase cost.

Significant portion of pharmacist working capital is tide up in inventory, i.e. small reduction in inventory gives more benefits like significant increase in working capital, decrease in amount of money needed to purchase further quantity.

Carrying cost includes specific items like insurance, taxes, interest, spoilage during handing, transport.

4 Differentiate between large volume parenterals and small volume parenterals.

☞ **Large Volume Parenterals (LVPs)**

1. LVPs are those parenterals having quantity equal to or more than 500 ml.
2. These are called infusions.
3. These are manufactured as single dose containers.
4. These are given by IV route.
5. Preservative is generally not needed.
6. For example, normal saline solution IP, BP USP, 5% dextrose infusion IP, BP.

These are used to provide nutrition, energy and as a drug carrier.

Small Volume Parenterals (SVPs)

1. SVPs are those parenterals having quantity near about 1 to 2 ml and maximum up to 40 ml.
2. These are called injections.
3. These are sometimes manufactured as multidose containers.
4. These can be given by IV as well as by other route.
5. Preservative is needed.
6. For example, adrenaline injection IP, BP.

These are used for treating diseases and also for prophylaxis purpose.

5 Enlist the facilities and requirements to be fulfilled for sterile manufacturing. (S. 09)

☞ For sterile manufacturing following equipment are necessary to satisfy the provisions of Drugs and Cosmetic Act, 1940.

(i) Hot air sterilizer
(ii) Cold storage and refrigeration unit
(iii) Autoclave
(iv) Labelling and packing unit
(v) Filter press
(vi) Sintered glass funnel
(vii) Filling and sealing unit
(viii) Seitz filter
(ix) Filter candles
(x) Storage for distilled water
(xi) Storage equipment for ampoules and vials
(xii) Ampoule washing machine
(xiii) Storage cabinets
(xiv) Water still
(xv) Leak testing unit.

6 Describe the layout of sterile product area. (S. 96, 01, 02; W. 96, 98, 01, 03, 06)

☞ The sterile manufacturing requires specific and particular areas for different purposes.

The product runs through these areas sequentially before it is finished.

These areas should be well coordinated with each other and areas should be free from microbial and particulate matter.

The sterile product areas can be subdivided as follows:

1. Clean up area
2. Preparation or compounding area
3. Aseptic area
4. Quarantine area
5. Finishing and packaging area
6. Service area
7. Quality control area
8. Office
9. Pre-entry washroom
10. Gowning area.

The floor plan of the sterile products area is given below:

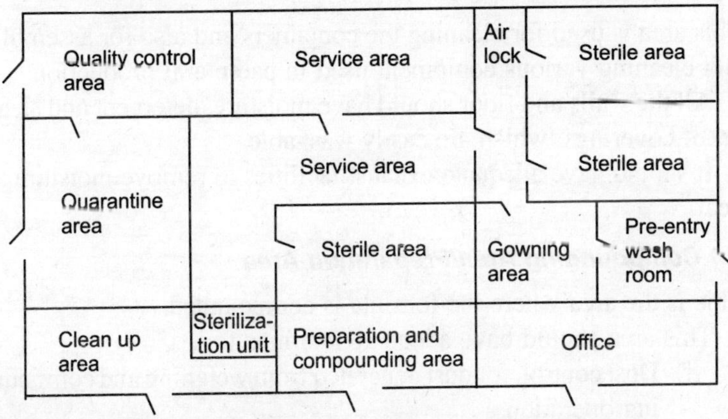

7 Give the ideal requirements/desirable properties of parenterals. Give the conditions to be fulfilled by all parenteral preparations. (S. 07, 09; W. 00)

☞ Ideal Qualities of Parenterals

1. It should be sterile.
2. It should be free from pyrogens.
3. It should be non-toxic and non-irritant.
4. It should be isotonic with body fluids.
5. It should be clear.
6. It should be free from foreign particles.

7. It should be chemically inert.
8. It should be free from inert gases.
9. It should be stable physically and chemically.
10. It should have a specific gravity similar to that of spinal fluid.

8 Write a note on production facility areas/production planning.

☞ Production area is divided into five sections:

(a) Clean up area.
(b) Compounding area/preparation area.
(c) Aseptic area/sterile area.
(d) Quarantine area.
(e) Packaging and labelling area.

(a) Clean up Area

This area is used for cleaning the containers and also for assembling and cleaning various equipment used in parenteral production.

All the walls and floor should have moisture, detergent and steam-proof coverings, which are easily washable.

It should have adequate exhaust facilities to remove moisture and heat.

(b) Compounding Area/Preparation Area

This is the area where the formula is compounded.

This area should have adequate facilities for:

(i) Dust control, for dust generated from weighing and compounding operations.
(ii) All cabinet and counters should be made of stainless steel.
(iii) All cabinets, cupboards and counters should be installed so that dirt does not accumulate.
(iv) Wall and floor coverings should be like clean up areas.

(c) Aseptic Area/Sterile Area (*S. 08*)

The area which is free form all microbes, dust particles is known as sterile area.

Design/Precautions/Construction/Requirements of Aseptic Area

1. Aseptic area should be away from crowdy area.
2. Windows must be provided with glass.

3. Laminar air flow should be provided.
4. The air in the aseptic area should be filtered through HEPA filter (high efficiency particulate air filters). This filter removes particles having diameter of 0.3 μm. This filter has 99.97% efficiency.
5. Doors should have air-lock system to prevent sudden rush of air inside.
6. Aseptic area should have positive pressure.
7. Ceiling walls and floors should be smooth and easily washable.
8. There should be minimum counters and should be made up of stainless steel.
9. Walls should have glazed tiles.
10. UV lamps should be provided to make air sterile.
11. All the equipment and apparatus should be sterilized.
12. The movements in the aseptic room must be minimum.
13. Sufficient space should be provided to the workers in aseptic area.
14. The person entering the room should enter through air-lock system and should wear sterile gown, cap, mask, gloves and footwares.
15. The person working in aseptic area should be free from any disease or disorder.
16. Regular medical check up of worker is necessary.

(d) Quarantine Area

In this area, the processed, sealed and tested products are kept for fixed duration and then again subjected for testing before sending then for labelling and packaging and marketing.

(e) Packaging and Labelling

Packaging should provide:

(i) Ample protection of the product against physical damage form handling and storage.
(ii) Should protect light-sensitive material form ultraviolet radiations.

Labelling: Labelling provides information needed to ensure safe and proper use of the therapeutic agent.

9 Write a note on "laminar air flow system." (S. 96, 97, 98, 01, 02, 05; W. 02, 06)

☞ Laminar Air Flow

"It is the cleaned air flow runs along parallel lines in confined area at a uniform velocity after having based through a HEPA filter."

This clean air sweeps contaminants away from the actual work area.

Two types of laminar flow systems are available depending on the direction of air flow.

1. Vertical laminar flow.
2. Horizontal laminar flow.

Preferred direction of air flow is vertical.

Laminar air flow principles have greatly improved the environmental control of aseptic areas.

For this purpose clean filtered aseptic air is blown evenly throughout the back of a hooded area or side of an entire room.

The air flow must be uniform in velocity and direction throughout any given cross-section of area being exhausted form opposite side.

The air velocity employed should be about 100 ft/ml.

Contamination is prevented because it sweeps away the air flow. Due to this environmental conditions are extremely good in both hooded work benches and entire room using laminar flow.

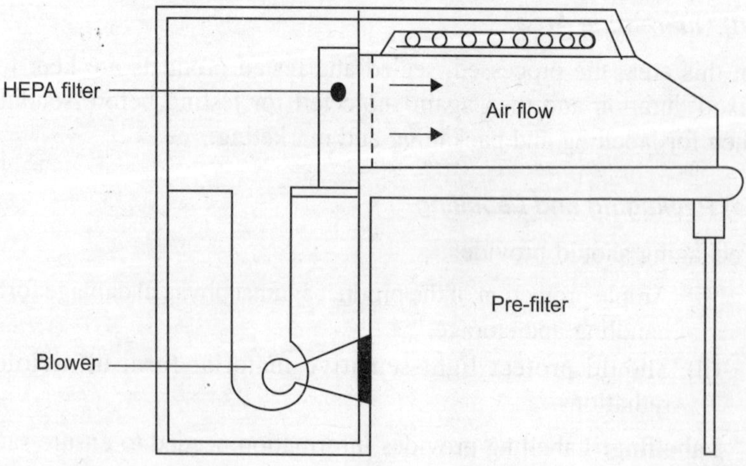

Laminar air flow bench

10 Explain various additives used in parenterals/injections. (S. 97, 05; W. 96, 02, 05)

☞ **Additives used in Parenterals**

1. **Vehicles:** Vehicle gives form and appearance to the parenteral preparations.
   Vehicles used in parenterals may be:
   (i) Aqueous vehicles, e.g. water for injection IP.
   - Purified water
   - Distilled water
   - Dextrose injection
   - Saline solution.

   (ii) Non-aqueous vehicle (oily), e.g. peanut oil, olive oil.
   (iii) Water miscible vehicle, e.g. ethyl alcohol, glycerin.
2. **Solubilizing agents:** These are necessary to increase the solubility of poorly water soluble drugs, e.g. twins, polysorbates.
3. **Stabilizers/antioxidants:** To prevent oxidation of product, antioxidants are added, e.g. tocopherols, BHT, BHA.
4. **Buffers:** Buffers are used to maintain pH of preparations, e.g. phosphate buffers and acetate buffers.
5. **Antimicrobial agents:** Bacteriostatic or fungistatic agents must be present in multidose containers to prevent growth of bacterial, etc.
6. **Tonicity contributors:** These are added to maintain isotonicity of the preparation, e.g. sodium chloride, borax, boric acid, dextrose.
7. **Wetting agents**, e.g. twins, sorbitol.
8. **Suspending agents**, e.g. acacia, methyl cellulose.
9. **Emulsifying agents**, e.g. lecithin.

11 Describe various stages/operations involved in manufacturing of parenterals or sterile dosage forms. (S. 01, W. 97, 00, 04)

☞1. **Washing and cleaning of containers, closures and equipment**

- All the containers, closures and equipment required in manufacturing of parenterals are thoroughly cleaned with the detergent and then washing with free flowing water followed by rinsing with water for injection.

- Finally they are dried and sterilized by suitable method.

2. **Collection of materials**
    - The materials required for formulation of parenteral preparations are weighed and collected in the preparation room.
    - All these materials must be of highest quality.
    - If water is vehicle, it should be free from pyrogens.
3. **Compounding and preparation:** For mixing and compounding standard procedures must be followed. The product should be compounded under clean environmental conditions.
4. **Filtration:** The solutions formed are then passed through a suitable filter medium to remove foreign particles. Bacteria-proof filters such as sintered glass filter, seitz filters are used for this purpose.
5. **Filling procedures:** After filtration and sterilization, the solutions are filled in the final containers like ampoules, vials and bottles.

    Bottle filling should be done by following methods:

    (i) Gravity filling.
    (ii) Pressure filling.
    (iii) Vacuum filling.
6. **Sealing of the containers**
    - Sealing of the containers should be done as early as possible to prevent the contamination of the product.
    - The rubber closures are fitted on the vials and bottles and sealed by crimping the aluminium cap which is done manually.
    - On small scale, the ampoules are sealed manually by rotating the neck of the ampoule in the flame of Bunsen burner to soften the glass which ultimately fuses to close the ampoule.
    - Sealing methods:

        (a) Tip sealing: Tip seals are made by melting sufficient glass at the tip of ampoule neck to form a bead of glass and close opening.

        (b) Pull sealing: Pull seals are made by healing the neck of a rotating ampoule below the tip, the pulling is always the up from a small twisted capillary just before being melted and closed.

7. Sterilization/terminal sterilization

- The sterilization of parenteral products in final containers is called terminal sterilization.
- Thermostable preparations are sterilized by autoclaving.
- Thermolabile preparations are sterilized by filtration and radiation.
- Only oily injections are sterilized by hot air oven.

8. Labelling and packaging

- All the containers, i.e. ampoules, vials, should be labelled properly with name, quantity, batch no., date of mfg, expiry, storage, retail price, manufacturer's address.
- Labelled container should be packed in a cardboard to avoid breakage during transportation.
- Ampoules should be packed in partition boxes.

9. Evaluation of parenterals: Stringent quality control of parenterals is necessary since they are introduced into the body directly. It should be done by quality control department by using following tests:

(i) Clarity test
(ii) Leaker test
(iii) Sterility test
(iv) Pyrogen test

12 Write a note on "procurement of stores". (S. 05, 08; W. 03) OR Write a procedure adopted by hospital pharmacist to procure drugs or hospital supplies.

☞ Store department in hospital is responsible for procurement of a number of things required to run a hospital successfully.

These purchases may be centralized for the entire hospital or may be decentralized by the respective departments, e.g. pharmacy.

Pharmacy procures drugs, medicines and essential goods used by clinical staff.

The procedure of purchasing is decided by PTC or by executive committee.

The purchasing material is classified as equipment and items of store. Pieces of equipment are machinery, apparatus, instruments, furniture, operation table, etc. Items of store include medicines, drugs, chemicals, surgical dressing materials, lab. reagents, etc.

The purchasing is done under a purchase medical officer. The source for purchasing is usually choosen from a licensed party with a good history, by pharmacists or the officer or by the purchase committee.

The method of purchasing includes:

(i) A direct purchase from wholesaler or manufacturers.
(ii) Quotations are invited for yearly supply.
(iii) Emergency purchases from local market.
(iv) Purchase by rate contract.

The purchasing involves two modern methods.

(a) Centralized Purchasing Method (S. 98, 00, 01; W. 00, 02, 08)

In this system, purchases are done for the entire hospital. All the items are purchased through a purchase committee at a time. Hence, called as centralized purchasing.

For this purpose requirement of each department of hospital is listed by head of every department and forwarded to purchasing committee.

The in-charge of this committee prepares consolidated and comparative statements. Further these statements are forwarded towards executive committee or governing body. This committee sanctions items which are to be purchased and such sanctioned items are listed by purchasing committee which were prepared in 7 copies. These copies are required for purchasing committee, audit department vendor, store, hospital administrator, governing body and related department.

(b) Decentralized Purchasing Method (S. 98, 00, 01, 08; W. 00, 02, 08)

If the purchases are done by individual department, it is called decentralized purchasing.

This method is useful for the goods like stationary, chairs, etc.
In this way the materials are procured for the store.

13 Describe to whom the copies of purchase orders are given and why? (S. 97, 00, 02, 09; W. 96, 00)

☞ The pharmacist is authorized to purchase on behalf of the clinical staff.

The copies (07) of purchase order are given to:

1st copy: Sent to supplier by post or hand delivery of supply.

2nd copy: Sent to accounts department where it will be retained for accounting.

3rd copy: Retained by purchasing officer for his department.

4th copy: Sent to the department from where request form is received.

5th copy: Completion of 5th copy is done if articles are received and sent to accounts department.

6th copy: It is utilized only when goods are back ordered.

7th copy: It is a specific copy kept by purchase officer for other use.

14 Discuss the following tests for parenterals/sterile dosage forms—(evaluation/quality control/pharmacopoeial tests/official tests). (S. 00; W. 08)

☞ A. Leaker Test

- Leaker test is carried out to detect capillary pores, cracks or incomplete seals in the ampoules.
- The ampoules are completely immersed in a dye solution (1% methylene blue) in a vacuum chamber.
- Vacuum is applied and is released after 10 minutes.
- If the seal is imperfect or a crack is observed, coloured solution enters into ampoules.
- This shows sample fails to pass leaker test.

B. Clarity Test

- Clarity test is used to detect presence of particulate matter in parenteral products.
- This test is useful only for solutions.
- In this test visual inspection of product (ampoule) is done against a black and white background in bright light.
- Transparent particles are visible against black background and coloured particles against white background.
- If visible particles are found in the sample then sample is found to be contaminated.

C. Sterility Test (S. 06)

- Principle: Sterility test is a technique used for checking the complete freedom from living microbes and their spores.
- Sterility test is based on the principle that if any contaminating bacteria or fungi present are placed in a nutrient medium under favorable conditions, it shows growth of microbes.

- The growth of microorganisms can be detected easily because clear medium turns turbid.

Official Methods of Sterility Testing

(a) Direct inoculation method (petridish/plate)

- A sterile petridish is taken and a sterile nutrient agar medium is added in it.
- The sample which is to be tested, is mixed with nutrient medium.
- Then the petridish is kept in incubator for 7 days under specified conditions.
- After 7 days, if turbidity appears, it is said that product is not sterile.

(b) Membrane filtration method

- In this method sample is filtered through a sterile membrane filter having porosity of 0.45 μm.
- After filtration membrane is washed with a sterile diluting fluid to remove traces of bacteriostatic agent.
- Then the membrane is aseptically removed and placed into a nutrient agar medium and incubated at 20°C for 7 days.
- The product passes the sterility test if no turbidity appears at the end of the incubation period.

D. Pyrogen Test (W. 08)

- Pyrogens are the metabolic products of living or dead microbes.
- Pyrogens cause rise in body temperature upon injection.
- The parenterals must be free from pyrogens.
- There are two methods of pyrogen testing.

(i) Biological Test (Using Rabbits)

- Rabbits are used for this test as they are highly sensitive to pyrogens.
- Three healthy rabbits are selected and suitable amount of sample is injected into the ear vein of the three rabbits.
- The rectal temperatures of all three rabbits are recorded.
- Any animal showing a rise in temperature of 0.6°C or more or if sum of the responses exceeds 1.4°C, then it indicates the presence of pyrogens in the parenteral preparations and vice versa.

Disadvantages or Limitations of Pyrogen Test

Using Rabbit Method

1. Healthy animals are required.
2. Animals show variation in their responses.
3. Influence of other factors may occur.
4. Some drugs cannot be tested satisfactorily because drug shows pharmacological action.
5. Time-consuming method.
6. Rectal thermometer with digital control is required.
7. Constant recording of temperature is necessary.
8. Sensitivity of test is less.

(ii) LAL Test/Bacterial Endotoxin Test (BET)

- It is based on the gelling of the reagent called limulus amoebocyte lysate (LAL) in the presence of bacterial endotoxins.
- Amoebocytes or the circulating blood cells of the horse-shoe crab contain a protein that clots in presence of pyrogens.
- If lyophilized (freeze dried) powder of LAL is added in the solution containing pyrogens it causes gel formation within 30 minutes.
- Thus in the test sample limulus amoebocyte lysate powder is added, if gelling appears, then it shows presence of pyrogens.

Advantages of LAL Test

1. Test is very simple.
2. It gives quick result.
3. Use of animals like rabbits is avoided.
4. Greater sensitivity than the rabbit test.
5. Very cheap method as it does not require equipments.

15 Name the methods used for sterilization of following:

☞ (i) Rubber gloves—γ-radiation, autoclaving, ethylene oxide.
(ii) Glasswares—Dry heat sterilization autoclaving.
(iii) Scalpel—Autoclave dry heat.
(iv) Transfusion/IV set—Ethylene oxide, γ-radiation.
(v) Plastic wound dressing—Ethylene oxide, γ-radiation.
(vi) Metal needles—Dry heat sterilization.
(vii) Glass syringe—Dry heat sterilization.
(viii) Absorbent cotton wool—Moist heat sterilization, γ-radiation.

(ix) Plastic wound dressing—Ethylene oxide, γ-radiation.

(x) Disposable syringes—γ-radiations, ethylene oxide.

NON-STERILE MANUFACTURING

16 Name the equipments required for manufacturing of tablet. What is non-sterile manufacture? (S. 97, 98, 99, 07; W. 98, 00, 02, 04)

☞ Non-sterile manufacture is the manufacture of preparations which do not require stringent sterility conditions while preparation and store as that of parenteral dosage forms.

Equipments for Manufacture of Tablets

1. Powder mixer, mass mixer
2. Disintegrator
3. Granulator
4. Oven
5. Tablet machine, single punch or rotary
6. Tablet counter
7. Coating pan
8. Exhaust system
9. Polishing pan
10. Heater.

17 What is general procedure for production of syrup? (S. 97, 03, 07; W. 00, 05, 06)

☞ **Hot Process**

This is the general method used for production of syrup when the active constituent is neither volatile nor heat sensitive.

The suitable amount of sucrose is weighed in a tared pan, purified water is added and heated on a water bath till a solution is obtained.

The product is strained and enough boiling purified water is added. Adjust the desired weight or volume, e.g. syrup IP, syrup of Tolu IP.

Other methods of preparation of syrup are:

(i) Percolation (cold process).

(ii) Agitation (without heat).

(iii) Addition of medicating liquid to syrup.

5

Pharmacy and Therapeutic Committee

1 What is pharmacy and therapeutic committee? Give composition/organization and operation of PTC. (S. 02, 04, 05, 06; W. 96, 99, 01, 02, 03, 06)

☞ PTC

PTC is a policy framing and recommending body on matters related to rational use of drugs in the hospital and consists of members from various departments of the hospital.

Composition of PTC

PTC consists of:

(i) At least 3 physicians
(ii) One nursing staff
(iii) One pharmacist (secretary)
(iv) Hospital administrator (chairman)

- Chairman is appointed from the physicians.
- Pharmacist is usually the secretary.
- There are approximately six meetings per year of the PTC.
- Secretary is responsible for preparation of agenda for meeting which should be submitted to all members well in advance.
- Secretary is also responsible for preparing minutes of the meeting.
- PTC is appointed by governing body/board of trustees.
- PTC is appointed for better control over routine services provided by hospital.

2 What are the two major objectives served by PTC? (S. 00, 03; W. 01)

☞ PTC serves following two main objectives:

(a) **Advisory:** It formulates the policies regarding selecting procuring, prescribing, dispensing and administering of drugs in a hospital.

It also consists of adaptation of policies providing suggestions to hospital staff and answering the queries asked by patients.

(b) **Educational:** It includes training of physicians, nurses, volunteers and pharmacists. PTC conducts various seminars to provide recent knowledge to physicians, nurses, pharmacists.

3 Describe the functions and scope of PTC. (S. 96, 97, 99, 00, 01, 04, 06; W. 98, 00, 02, 03, 04, 05, 06, 08)

☞ **Functions of PTC**

1. It develops policies regarding drug safety.
2. It develops hospital formulary system.
3. It promotes rational use of drugs without wastage and duplication of drugs.
4. It takes review of hospital formulary.
5. It provides training to physicians, nurses, volunteers.
6. It develops policies and procedures for the purchasing, distribution, selection and storage and uses of drugs.
7. It manages the educational programmes for hospital staff.
8. It gives advice to pharmacy department about the purchasing, storage of the dugs and medicinal products.
9. It plays an effective role in hospital management and can prepare subcommittee for purchasing, maintenance, etc.
10. It inspects over the routine activities of the hospital.
11. It partly controls over the hospital library.
12. It gives different suggestions to manufacturing department of the hospital.
13. It can also take decisions about 'automatic stop order' for the dangerous drugs or for the drugs showing unwanted effects.
14. It makes the list of emergency drugs, dangerous drugs, narcotic drugs, alcohol containing and other drugs.
15. It interacts with FDA department.

16. It promotes rational use of drugs.
17. It gives guidelines regarding addition and deletion of drugs in hospital.
18. It helps to review ADR in hospital.
19. It decides quality norms for distribution, administration and use of medication.
20. It advises the pharmacy in procedures for effective drug distribution and control procedures.

4 Explain the role of PTC in drug safety. OR How does PTC ensure drug safety in hospital? (S. 05, 07, 08; W. 97)

☞ Drug safety is one of the major responsibilities of the hospital pharmacist.

The PTC can play an effective role in ensuring drug safety on a continuous basis, by creating safety awareness in all departments of the hospital.

For drug safety in hospital, PTC should consider following points during its administration.

1. Employment of qualified person as a 'chief pharmacist' (B Pharm) and rest are diploma holders.
2. Takes care that the medicines are dispensed only by pharmacists.
3. Sufficient number of pharmacists are employed to cover full day in different shifts of 8 hours.
4. Proper adequate storage facilities are to be provided in pharmacy.
5. Drugs classified under poisons are stored separately from non-poisonous drugs.
6. Stock and issue of narcotic and psychotic substances shall confirm to legal requirements.
7. Follow of GMP effectively in manufacturing section.
8. External preparations are kept separately and dispensed in special containers, which are distinctively different form the liquid orals like syrups and mixtures.
9. Empty infusion glass bottles (saline bottles) should never be permitted for other uses like collection to urine, vomits, bringing coffee and storing of antiseptic solutions.

10. Physical verification taken to remove expired drugs, deteriorated drugs.
11. Providing a library and documentation facility.
12. Conducting lectures, seminars on modern methods of dispensing to staff of the hospital.
13. For effective functioning, PTC forms several subcommittees like subcommittee for narcotic drugs, for CNS drugs, for CVS agents, for GIT agents, for neoplastic agents, etc.

6

Hospital Formulary

1 What is hospital formulary? What is the aim or need of hospital formulary system? (S. 96, 97, 00, 02, 03, 04, 05; W. 97, 98, 99, 01)

☞ Hospital Formulary

It is continuously revised collected information of pharmaceutical dosage forms which gives current clinical judgement to the medical staff.

It is continuously revised compilation of pharmaceutical dosage forms.

Aims/Need of Hospital Formulary

1. To provide best possible treatment to the patients in lowest possible cost is the ultimate aim served by a hospital formulary.
2. It informs the physicians, nurses and pharmacists about the new and more potent drugs available in the hospital.
3. It avoids the use of brand and therapeutic duplication of drugs.
4. It promotes rational use of drugs.
5. To provide guidelines for 'procuring, prescribing, dispensing and administering of drugs in a hospital'.
6. It informs about availability of medicines, dosage forms and their quantity in the hospital.
7. To inform the staff about standard dosage regimen, adverse effects of the drugs.
8. It provides guidelines regarding emergency drugs in a hospital.

9. It contains list of physicians, their address, phone numbers, qualification and available timings in the hospital which is useful for reference or in emergency conditions.
10. It informs the staff about reported ADRS in the hospital.

2 Write guidelines for hospital formulary system. OR Explain guidelining principles of HPS. (S. 96, 05, 06; W. 97, 98, 08)

☞ 1. It provides policies, procedures for purchasing and distribution of medicines.
2. It provides information to nursing staff about doses, uses, route of administration of the drugs.
3. It provides information and guidelines about dispensing of medicines and maintenance of documents to pharmacist.
4. It provides information about manufacturing, repacking and labelling of medicines.
5. It provides information to the physicians about available drugs in the hospital along with their quantity.
6. It provides guidelines regarding maintenance of stock of medicine for the pharmacist.
7. It is useful for preparation of purchase list, purchase order, checking of stock to the pharmacist.

3 Explain the significance/functions/importance/role of hospital formulary system. (S. 97, 98, 01, 02, 03, 04, 06; W. 98)

☞ 1. It provides greatest benefits to the patients and physicians (therapeutic).
2. It eliminates duplication of drugs thus reducing inventory duplication.
3. It gives prescribing tips and additional drug information.
4. It provides current and modern developments in medicines.
5. It helps in evaluating and selecting drugs in the hospitals.
6. It gives guidelines regarding prescribing, procuring, dispensing and administering of a drugs in hospital.
7. The information in the hospital formulary is useful for physicians, nurses, pharmacists in the hospital.
8. It provides availability of stock of drugs in the hospital.

9. It gives information about reported adverse reactions in the hospital and hence staff should take care to avoid further possibilities of ADRs.
10. It also contains list of emergency drugs, poisonous drugs, etc.
11. It contains aims and objectives of the hospital.
12. It contains list of physicians, qualification and their available timings so that other staff and patients may get benefited.
13. HFS also informs about use of drug, precautions, contraindication of the drugs and doses of drugs.

4 Give the format of hospital formulary/what is the nature of hospital formulary/give the formate and contents of HF. (S. 07, 08, 09; W. 04)

☞ Contents of HF

It contains:

1. Pharmacological index
2. Alphabetical index of drugs.
3. List of emergency drugs.
4. List of narcotic drugs, dangerous drugs, etc.
5. List of drugs with their uses, doses and dosage forms, route of administration, precautions, contraindications, and adverse reactions, etc.
6. List of physicians with their address, phone numbers, qualification and available timings at the hospital.
7. Current developments, research in pharmacy and medical field.
8. Information about addition and deletion of drugs.
9. Reported ADRs in the hospital.

Format of HF

- Format of hospital formulary is decided by PTC.
- Generally, it should be in binded form.
- The size of HF is decided by PTC.
- It should be light in weight, easy to carry.
- It should contain minimum but essential information.
- The coloured pages are not allowed.
- It should contain any advertisement.
- Only white paper and black ink is allowed for preparation of HF.

5 How is hospital formulary prepared?

☞ Hospital is devised by pharmacy and therapeutic committee.

- Pharmacist is an important member of this committee.
- PTC takes decision about addition and deletions of drugs.
- After that, pharmacist edit the information and undertakes the production, printing and complication, etc. of formulary.
- Once it is decided to have formulary, the contents other than drugs included are also to be decided, e.g. prescription writing, use of drugs, diagnostic agents, toxicology section, posology, useful tables/data.
- The pharmacist is informed of all these decisions. The preparation of a formulary is then a routine production function.

6 How are entry (addition) and deletion of drugs in the hospital formulary done? (W. 96, 06)

☞ The decisions of addition and deletion of drugs in HF are taken by PTC.

Addition/Entry of a Drug into HF

For addition of any drug into hospital following things should be considered:

1. The drug should be well accepted in market or otherwise should have 'No objection certificate' from FDA under the D & C Act.
2. The drug should have sufficient 'margin of safety', i.e. minimum side effects and good pharmacological action with minimum dose.
3. Marketed products should mention their license no., registration no., address of registered office of the company and essential information about the medicine.
4. PTC checks the information about drug and the effects of drugs should be monitored and then through discussions and seminars PTC informs the physicians about the use of drugs.
5. After confirming effectivity of drug PTC permits the particular drug to enter into the hospital pharmacy.

Deletion of the Drugs from HF

The ADR/drug interaction/unwanted side effect if observed with patient then it should be reported by physicians to PTC.

The information regarding ADRs should be reported to PTC by following type of form:

ADRs

Date:	Time:
Dosage form:	Name of the drug:
Patient's name:	Age: Sex:

Type of disease:

Observed side effects/ADR/Interaction:

Other information:

Signature of Applicant

The PTC calls meeting and the physicians should show the ADRs of the drug through seminar and discussion. After that PTC decides the deletion of a particular drug.

7

Drug Information Service and Drug Information Bulletin

1 What do you know about drug information service/ centre? Give the need/objectives of DIS/DIC. What are the abilities of a person required to run DIS/DIC? (S. 96, 00, 01, 02, 03, 05; W. 98, 99, 00, 01)

☞ **DIS/DIC**

"Drug information centre is one of the departments of the hospital and gives the recent knowledge and information about the medical, pharmacy field at any time to the physicians, staff of the hospital and to the citizens."

NEED of DIC

1. To give first aid suggestions.
2. To get knowledge about recent developments in medical and supportive services.
3. To get idea about emergency treatments.
4. To clarify the queries about medical and supportive fields.
5. To store the information and retrieve it.
6. For adjustment of better drug therapy.
7. To provide vital and necessary information to physicians and medical persons.

Abilities/Qualities required by a Pharmacist to run DIS/DIC (S. 97, 98)

DIS/DIC should be run by pharmacist who should have following abilities:

1. He should be able to edit the information.
2. He can collect the data, quickly and accurately.
3. He should have good communication skills.
4. He should have a knowledge about research method and about the sources of information.
5. He should have knowledge about medical, pharmacy and nursing field.
6. He should attend the seminars, conferences and should collect essential information.
7. He should have an ability to study obstracts, literatures, journals and also should be able to deliver the knowledge to others.
8. He is the member of PTC and should have a knowledge about various aspects of drugs.

2 Give the location, requirements and facilities required for drug information centre/DIS.

☞ Location of DIS/DIC

- It should be away from inpatient department and should be possibly away from outpatient department also.
- This department should be near to pharmacy department and also near to the hospital library.
- It should provide essential environment for reading the books. Thus, it should be having negligible disturbances.

Requirements and Facilities of DIC

1. This department should provide good furniture, adequate books, audiovisual arrangements for conduction of seminars, photocopy, e-mail, fax, computers, telephones.
2. It should provide adequate electric and water facilities.
3. This centre should have rectangular, circular tables and adequate chairs.
4. The dimensions of this centre are dependant on size of hospital, type of hospital, number of staff utilizing library, number of publications to be kept in and overall utilization by citizens.
5. The reading area provided to the reader should be minimum 25 to 30 sq. feet. The minimum distance between two tables

should be at least 5 feet and the distance in between wall and table should not be less than 3 feet.

6. It should have official books like several pharmacopoeias, remingtons pharmaceutical sciences, national formulary, various journals (American Journal of Hospital Pharmacy, Journal of Pharmacognosy, Indian Journal of Medical Research).
7. This dept. should be open for 24 hours.
8. It should have facility to conduct seminars for giving recent knowledge to the staff.

3 Write the functions of DIC/DIS.

☞ Functions of DIC

1. **Collection and storage of information:** By reading the obstracts, journals, periodicals, the head of this centre obtains information and store it in the computers.
2. **Retrieval of information:** Whenever required the information is read by staff of hospital to get knowledge of recent development and to clarify queries.
3. **Evaluation of information:** The information is read by head of this centre and edited by him and published in drug information bulletin.
4. **As a community centre:** This centre communicate with other hospitals and arrange the seminars, lectures in that community to increase the educational standard of the public. If also clears the queries asked by citizens, therefore, increases the status of the hospital.
5. **As an information center:** It provides information about emergency treatment, first aid treatment and also about poisons and toxic substances.
6. **Information for research:** This department provides information to the staff involved in research work.
7. **Information regarding reported ADRs:** This department provides information regarding reported ADRs to other hospitals so that further ADRs do not occur.
8. This department has facilities like fax, e-mail, telephone therefore, quick information can be collected by citizens.
9. It is opened for 24 hours for getting the information.

4 What is drug information bulletin? Explain DIB. (S. 07; W. 97, 98, 99, 01, 02)

☞ **DIB**

It is the bulletin printed and published by DIC of the hospital which contains latest developments in medical science, new drugs introduced, update of drug interactions and adverse drug reactions.

Contents of DIB

1. It contains recent information about the drugs, developments and dosage forms.
2. It contains information about new methods of analysis, services offered by the hospitals, any ADRs reported in the hospital.
3. Question-answer type section.
4. Puzzles.
5. Latest information about developments in medical, paramedical services.
6. It should be published by hospital for internal circulation only.
7. The information in bulletin is collected and edited by the head of PTC.
8. This bulletin contains names of reference books, journals, proceedings of conferences.

Sources of Information

The sources of information for DIB are as follows:

(a) **Primary sources:** It contains the information published by authority and it is generally called raw information. This information is nothing but articles in journals, obstracts, etc.

(b) **Secondary sources:** It contains the comments or opinions or modified information. The information is collected from pharmacopoeias formulary textbooks, etc. This information is evaluated by second party, i.e. original information is selected, modified, rearranged and condensed.

(c) **Tertiary sources:** These are outputs of primary and secondary sources.

***Importance/Need/Significance of DIB* (*W. 96, 99, 01*)**

1. It is the link between DIC and other health professionals.
2. It is the way of communication for giving the information to the physicians, pharmacist and also within very short time.
3. It is important for keeping the medical staff of hospital alert about the recent knowledge and developments.
4. A regular publication of the bulletin will update the knowledge of the patient care staff on the development in their area of specialization.

8

Computers in Hospital Pharmacy

1 Define computer. Give merits and demerits of computer. Explain its role in hospital pharmacy.

☞ Computer

"It is the electric device performing the several complex and complicated functions and can store the information."

Advantages/Merits

1. High speed
2. Storage capacity—softwares, floppy disc, hard disc
3. Easy retrieval of data
4. Accurate results
5. Can perform complicated, several arithmetical and logical functions
6. Time saving
7. Space saving
8. Economic
9. Can work for 24 hours.

Disadvantages/Demerits

1. Cannot correct itself.
2. Lack of common sense.
3. Depends upon human instructions.
4. Electricity is required.
5. Skilled person is required for operation.

Role of Computers in Hospital Pharmacy

Computers are used more frequently for wide variety of work in hospital pharmacy.

1. In drug store for billing, purchasing, stocking, ordering, etc.
2. In hospital pharmacy to record prescriptions.
3. In pathological laboratory.
4. In manufacturing section of hospital pharmacy.
5. In maintenance of patients' records.
6. In data storage and retrieval.
7. In inventory control.
8. In medication order entry.
9. In drug therapy monitoring.
10. In reporting ADRs.
11. In purchasing and accounting.
12. In billing of charge floor stock.

2 Describe in brief different parts/components of computer.

☞ The basic components of computer are:

1. CPU (central processing unit)
2. Monitor
3. Keyboard.

(i) CPU

It is the main component in which data is processed.

The capacity of hard disc depends upon total number of microprocessor units.

CPU consists of two types of memories:

1. RAM [Random assess memory]
2. ROM [Read only memory]

RAM is volatile, i.e. remains assist even if computer is off.

CPU has three drives and each drive has three connections.

(a) To main switch.

(b) To display unit.

(c) To keyboard.

In CPU, the input is analyzed, evaluated and processed and the output can be displayed on monitor.

CPU has 2 drives for insertion of floppies called drive A and B. The separate drive for CD is available.

(ii) Monitor

It is also called display unit or VDU. It has 3 buttons for brightness, contrast and on-off button.

It has two connections, i.e. to CPU and main suitch. Display capacity is 25 rows and 50 columns.

Monitor may be coloured or black and white.

(iii) Keyboard and Mouse

It is a commonly used input device. It is available in 2 types:

(a) 84 keyboard

(b) 101 keyboard.

It has alphabetical, functional, numerical and specific keys. 84 type keyboard has 10 functional keys while 101 type has 12 functional keys. Keyboard is connected to CPU only.

Mouse: Mouse is input device whenever required.

3 How are computers useful in record maintenance? (S. 96, 00, 01, 02, 04; W. 97, 99, 05, 06)

☞ Records in hospital pharmacy can be conveniently grouped as:

1. Records related to patient.
2. Records related to drug.

1. **Records related to patient:** It includes:

(a) Personal information of the patient like:

Name:	Occupation:	Date of admission:
Age:	Address:	Date of transfer:
Sex:	Ward no:	Date of discharge:
	Bed no:	

(b) Drug allergies and habits and diseases, etc:

Allergies:	Non-prescribe drug:
Body disorders:	Addicted by:
Previous disorders:	

2. **Records related to drugs prescribed to the patient on daily basis**

Date:	Route of administration:
Name of drug:	Frequency of drug administration:
Dose of drug:	Changes in dose of drug:

3. Records related to charges or bill to the patient for charged floor drugs.
4. Records related to ADRs if reported.
5. Inventory control record for drugs in hospital formulary.

Date base is collection of information related with particular section in hospital. MEDLINE is loaded in computer, which is a medical literature data base. It helps to mention medical records and also for taking the correct decisions about the diagnosis and treatment.

Data of physicians like name, qualification, address, phone no, are stored in computers so that emergency contact is possible. Prescriptions can be recorded and stored in computers so that patient compliance, refilling frequency can be checked.

PAD, MEDIPHORS, MEDLARS packages related to drug information are available which are useful in hospital pharmacy department. For maintenance of records of employees computer is useful. The names, qualification, experience, payments, allowances and other information are also maintained.

4 Define drug inventory. Explain the role of computers in inventory control. (S. 96, 97, 98, 03, 09; W. 00, 04)

☞ Drug Inventory

"Drug inventory control is a balance between not ordering too much and avoiding out-of-stock situation."

There are two types of systems used in inventory control:

1. Periodic inventory control system
2. Perpetual system.

Role of Computers in Inventory Control and Purchasing

In inventory control, computer is useful to maintain the records of inventory, distribution or available stock. For preparing budget and for statistical analysis separate packages are available in market. By taking these packages inventory control can be performed.

Computers show minimum and maximum stock levels and also reorder levels so that requirements and purchase order can be prepared.

1. **Periodic inventory control system:** In this system one person is appointed to check the stock of items periodically so that no extra items are stocked and it avoids inventory.

2. **Perpetual system:** In this method day to day checking of stock and checking of store ledger is done which gives correct information regarding actual stock at hand. Thus, further purchasing procedure can be started.

The main use of computers in purchase and inventory control is:

(i) To detect the items which have reached minimum order level.
(ii) To prepare list of items to be purchased and their quantities.
(iii) To prepare purchase order for vendors and avoids duplication of orders.
(iv) To detect infrequently purchased items for possible return or elimination from pharmacy drug supply.
(v) To produce periodic summary and purchasing and inventory control statistic.
(vi) Inventory control of drugs manages current stocks, outgoing stocks, incoming stocks, order procedure, etc.

5 Explain the role of computers in medication monitoring or in monitoring of drugs in hospitalized patients. (S. 99, 03, 05; W. 04)

☞ Medication Monitoring

It means constant supervision by pharmacist on the administered drugs to the patients to observe the specific pharmacological action, drug-interaction or adverse effects if any.

For monitoring of drugs computers provide immediately statistical data of drugs and also show variations in pharmacological actions as the doses administered, e.g. in cardiac patients changes in pulses, heartbeats, etc.

(i) Computers generate hourly 'fill lists' of drugs for patient and pharmacist prepares and dispense unit dose for each patient along with proper label and sends this for administration of drugs to the patient.
(ii) Prior to this, check is made for drug to drug interaction.
(iii) Medication administered in ward to the patient is entered in computer as medicine administration record.
(iv) Drug lab-test values are also recorded if required.

This cycle continues till the time patient is hospitalized. For monitoring drug therapy hand-held computer terminals can be used by clinical pharmacist on hospital floor or at the patient's bedside.

These terminals have sophisticated programs for predicting drug levels and required dosing parameter based on pharmacokinetic principles.

To maximize the therapeutic action of the drugs and avoiding any toxic effects, pharmacist starts taking help of some pharmacokinetic and non-pharmacokinetic parameters. This method of therapeutic drug monitoring is most important in geriatric and pediatric patients.

Thus in medication monitoring computer will have mainly two types of applications:

(a) **Pharmacokinetic applications:** It includes statistical calculation and graphical interpretations. By using computer programs like NONLIN the pharmacokinetic parameters can be predicted very easily. Depending on these parameters dose of drug administration can be adjusted.

(b) **Non-pharmacokinetic applications:** It includes drug-drug, drug-laboratory, drug-allergy, drug-disease interaction detection.

6 Explain how computers are useful in data storage and retrieval. (S. 99; W. 96, 98, 00)

☞ • Various softwares like MEDLAR, AMA, FOOD ID, MEDIPHOR, PAD, etc. are available in the market.

- These softwares contain the information about drugs, their description, uses, doses, side effects, dosage forms, etc.
- Packages like MEDIPHOR means monitoring and evaluation of drug interaction by pharmacy oriented reporting system which contains information about drug interaction.
- Other package like AMA means American Medical Association and contains description and diagnostic symptoms for more than 3500 diseases and information of special cases.
- These packages provide the information therefore, whenever required this information can be retrieved and therefore, further useful for research work and record keeping.
- Whenever required the information about the physiological parameters, properties of drug, pharmacological actions is used to develop new drugs or its dosage form. For this QUAR package is useful.
- In computer the data of patients such as name, age, sex, address, patient history, case papers, report of analysis, diagnosis papers, drug therapy given can be stored. Therefore, record keeping is easier.

- Due to retrieval facility the information is used to study refilling frequency, patient compliance, to make drug history and to send reminder to the patient.

7 Explain the role of computers in pathology laboratory.

☞ The packages like LNS, KINPAK, NONLIN, SUMEX are loaded on computers therefore, analysis reports can be obtained quickly with probable diagnosis.

Simultaneously reports are stored in computers therefore, documentation will be easier.

The paper work is also minimized.

Whenever required, information can be stored and retrieved.

8 Explain the role of computers in drug store. (S. 00, 07, 08)

☞ Computers have several advantages like more speed, great accuracy, and more working power, negligible mistakes, storage of information, etc. Therefore, they are used in drug store for:

1. Maintenance of records
2. Preparing purchase list
3. Preparing purchase order
4. For budget adjustment
5. Preparation of receipt
6. Storage of prescriptions
7. To prepare a list of expired drugs
8. To control overstocking and understocking of drugs
9. To get information of different manufacturers, their products, brand names and prices, etc.
10. It helps to prepare comparative statement of questions from different suppliers/manufacturers.

9 Explain the applications of computers in hospitals. (S. 06; W. 03)

☞ In hospitals a number of departments are present. As per requirements the computers can be used for getting several types of applications. In hospitals computers have wide scope in following departments.

1. Drug information centre
2. Pharmacy department

3. Manufacturing section
4. Clinical pharmacy department
5. Consulting section
6. Registration counter
7. Billing and accounting section.

In all these departments computers help to store so much information and avoids paper work.

It also helps in diagnosis of various disorders, medication, monitoring, etc.

It helps in charging of the prescription for charged floor stock.

For DIC it is very important to collect, edit the information for registration of the patient it helps and to take basic information of the patient and store it in a particular file.

Part II
Clinical Pharmacy

9

Introduction to Clinical Pharmacy

1 Define clinical pharmacy. Give its objectives. (S. 99, 04, 05, 09; W. 06, 08)

☞ **Definition**

1. Clinical pharmacy is a part of hospital pharmacy which deals with the preparation of patient drug profiles, recording patient drug history, advise about possible drug-drug interactions to trainees and drug effects on clinical laboratory test results.
2. Clinical pharmacy is a new-born discipline that carries a traditional hospital pharmacist from product-oriented approach to healthier patient-oriented approach, so as to ensure the patient's maximum well-being, while on drug therapy.

Objectives of Clinical Pharmacy

1. To assist the physicians in doing a better job of prescribing and monitoring drug therapy.
2. To assist nurses in administering medications (drugs).
3. To increase the patients' role in drug use process.
4. To maximize the effectiveness of drug therapy with minimum side effects or adverse effects.
5. To decrease the patients' non-compliance through the patient counseling.
6. To study drug therapy by monitoring it and it should maintain the records of drug therapies, any adverse effect or drug

interaction should be reported to the PTC of hospital and also to physician of the hospitals.

2 Discuss the role/scope/functions of clinical pharmacy/clinical pharmacist. (S. 96, 97, 98, 00, 01, 02, 03, 04, 05, 07, 09; W. 96, 97, 98, 00, 01, 02, 03, 05, 06)

☞ 1. Preparation of history of patient.
2. Preparation of drug history.
3. Participation in management of medical emergency.
4. Participation in drug investigation.
5. Participation in the management of chronic diseases like diabetes, hypertension, arthritis.
6. To control over drug utilization.
7. To monitor drug therapy.
8. To counsel with patient.
9. To help in selection of drug therapy to physician.
10. To communicate with physician and nurses through presentation and publication.
11. Detection and reporting of adverse drug reactions (ADRs).
12. To take part in educational programme related with medical pharmacy and nursing profession.
13. To provide the formal and informal consultation to the physician.
14. To explain the direction of use, route of administration and other related information to the patients.
15. Collection of knowledge of drug therapy and pharmacokinetics of drugs.
16. To take part in patients education, vaccination programme and other programmes related to social welfare arranged by the hospital.

3 What are the abilities required for clinical pharmacist?

Abilities of Clinical Pharmacist

☞ 1. He should have basic skill of the communication.
2. He should know about drug profile and pathophysiology of drug.
3. He should have advanced knowledge about pharmacology, pharmacokinetics and biopharmaceutics.
4. He should have adequate patience and better interest for development of clinical pharmacy.

5. He should have an interest in patient care.
6. He should have an art of giving information to the physician.
7. He should have knowledge of drug-drug interactions and adverse drug reactions.

4 What are the barriers in the development of clinical pharmacy?

☞ Barriers in the Development of Clinical Pharmacy

1. Lack of knowledge.
2. Lack of motivation.
3. Lack of vocational courses.
4. Lack of inter- and intraprofessional discussions.
5. Lack of self-confidence.
6. Lack of multidisciplinary approach.
7. Lack of team approach.
8. Confusion about the role of clinical pharmacist.
9. The clinical pharmacy practice is supposed to be an encroachment by the physicians.

5 What steps should be taken in the development of clinical pharmacy? (W. 08)

☞ 1. Hospital pharmacist should increase the need of clinical pharmacist by performing counseling with patient and physician.
2. Hospital pharmacist should increase the knowledge and should be involved in interprofessional discussions.
3. Government should start different vocational courses related to clinical pharmacy.
4. Pharmacist should clarify the querries asked by physician and patient.
5. Pharmacist should increase the necessity of clinical pharmacist.
6. Pharmacist and physicians should have a team approach in taking care of the patients.
7. Pharmacist should understand exact role of clinical pharmacist.

10

Modern Aspects of Dispensing

1 What is patient compliance? Explain factors influencing (affecting) patient compliance. (S. 03, 06; W. 00, 01, 04, 08)

☞ **Patient Compliance**

"A faithful adherence by the patient to the prescriber's instructions about rest, diet, exercise and drug therapy is called patient compliance."

- The term 'patient compliance' suggests that the patient does not follow the instructions given by physician about appropriate use of medications.
- The percentage of patient compliance can be calculated as follows:

$$\text{Percentage patient compliance} = \frac{\text{NPD} - \text{NME}}{\text{NPD}} \times 100$$

Where, NPD = Number of prescribed doses.
NME = Number of medication errors.

Factors Influencing/Affecting Patient Compliance

1. **Type of disease:** The patients suffering from acute diseases have more compliance than patients having chronic diseases.
2. **Age of the patient:** Elder patients always show more compliance than the aged patients.
3. **Duration of drug therapy:** The patients on short-term therapy show more compliance than on long-term therapy.

4. **Family background:** The patients who live alone show less patient compliance than patients who live with their families.
5. **Type of patients:** Inpatients show more compliance than outpatients.
6. **Frequency of drug administration:** The patients follow instruction when frequency of administration is less, i.e. more the frequency of administration of drug, lesser is the compliance.
7. **Side effects of drug therapy:** The patients if suffering from side effects of the drug therapy then discontinuation of drug may decrease the patient compliance.
8. **Cost of medication:** More the cost of medication lesser the patient compliance.
9. **Educational status:** Uneducated patients show less compliance than educated ones.

2 What is patients non-compliance? Explain the factors Influencing/affecting non-compliance. OR What are the causes/reasons for non-compliance? (S. 06)

☞ Patients Non-compliance

"Patients non-compliance refers to the error, faults or failure by the patient for following the instructions about the drug therapy, diet, exercise and rest, etc."

Factors Affecting/Influencing Patients Non-compliance

1. **Type of disease:** The patients suffering from chronic disease show more non-compliance as compared to those suffering from acute diseases.
2. **Age of the patient:** Younger patients show non-compliance than elder patient.
3. **Duration of therapy:** Patient on long-term therapy shows more non-compliance than on short-term therapy.
4. **Family background:** The patients who live alone show more non-compliance than patients who live with their families.
5. **Type of patient:** Outpatients show more non-compliance than inpatients.
6. **Frequency of drug administration:** If frequency of drug administration is more then patient shows non-compliance.

7. **Side effects of the drugs:** If the patient suffers from any side effect from the drug then he stops the doses of drug which gives rise to non-compliance.
8. **Cost of medication:** (Economic status of the patient) more the cost of medication greater is the non-compliance.
9. **Educational status:** Uneducated patients show more non-compliance than educated ones.
10. **Patient-pharmacist/patient-physician interaction:** Language, cultural or other communication barriers result into inadequate transfer of information about medication to patient by doctor or pharmacist and thus may show patient non-compliance.

3 What is the role of pharmacist to improve patient compliance? OR What is the role of pharmacist to decrease patient non-compliance?

☞ The pharmacist plays an important role in improving patient compliance:

1. The pharmacist should counsel the patient about the instruction given by physician about the rest, diet, exercise and drug therapy.
2. He should clarify querries/doubts asked by the patient.
3. He should motivate the patient to follow the instruction given by prescriber.
4. He should provide the knowledge to the patient about the disorders or diseases which the patient is suffering from.
5. He should discuss with the patient about his economical status and family background by asking some direct and indirect questions.
6. He should collect information about the habits and way of thinking of the patient.
7. He should provide knowledge about the drug therapy by considering the allergies, habits and body disorders of the patients.
8. He should inform the patient about the main drug, supplementary drug, mechanism of actions of drugs.
9. He should tell to the patient about the side effects of the drug and also about the refilling frequency of drug therapy.

10. He should also tell to the patient about the timing of administration, dose, frequency and route of administration of drug and any interaction with food.
11. He should increase patients involvement in drug use process and thus he can increase the patient compliance.
12. He should also discuss with the patient about the consequences of under or over utilization of drugs.
13. He should adjust drug therapy by use of minimum drugs with maximum beneficial effects.

In this way pharmacist helps to improve patient compliance.

4 Define patient counselling. Write the role of pharmacist in patient counselling. (S. 98, 03, 07; W. 96, 97, 01, 03, 04, 05, 06, 08)

☞ Patient Counselling

"Patient counselling is the part of clinical pharmacy practice to give maximum benefits to the patient and includes the instruction or advice given by the pharmacist to the patient about the use of the drugs prescribed."

Counselling should include following titles:

1. **How to remove the drug from the package:** If it is found that patient is not familiar with packaging the pharmacist should demonstrate how to remove the medicine form the package.
2. **Route of administration:** Pharmacist should tell the patient about route by which medicine should be taken, e.g. by mouth, to be instilled into eye, ear, or to be rubbed on the skin.
3. **Time of drug administration:** The pharmacist should instruct the patient about the time of administration of drug, e.g. every 6 hours, at bed time.
4. **Duration of drug therapy:** The pharmacist must ensure that the patient understands clearly the length of time, the medication is to be used. Otherwise resistance may develop.
5. **Storage of drugs:** The pharmacist should counsel the patient about the proper storage of the medicine to ensure safety and stability. Medicines should be beyond the reach of children at home.

6. **Side effects of drugs:** Possible side effects should be told tactfully to the patient.
7. **Drug interactions:** The patient should be warned about drug interaction which mainly occurs with food, e.g. tetracyclines with milk.
8. **Allergies:** Pharmacist should ask the patient about drug allergies to him to avoid further complications.
9. **Refilling frequency:** Pharmacist should indicate whether or not the prescription is refillable or should be refilled.
10. **About therapeutic effects of drugs:** Pharmacist should tell the patient about effectivity and use of drug.
11. Pharmacist should advise the patient about rest, diet and exercise.

Significance of Patient Counselling

1. It gives maximum benefits to the patient.
2. It avoids adverse effects of the drugs.
3. It avoids drug-food interactions.
4. It improves patient compliance.
5. Patient can understand safe and appropriate use of medicines.
6. It avoids over utilization and underutilization of drugs.

5 What are the consequences of under- or overutilization of drugs?

☞ Underutilization of Drugs

Underutilization of drugs means administration of low quantity of medicines.

Underutilization includes omitting the dose, insufficient quantity of dose is taken, missing of doses, failure in refilling of doses, failure in consumption of any one of prescribed drugs.

The consequences due to underutilization are dependant on types of drug, type of drug history, type of disease, pharmacological action of drug and body disorder of the patient, e.g.

1. Propranolol, clonidine are hypotensive drugs. Omition of dose of these drugs causes rebound hypertension.
2. Phenytoin, phenobarbitone are antiepileptic drugs. Missing of doses of these drugs may cause rebound epileptic attacks which are severe than previous ones.

3. Underutilization of antitubercular drugs may produce drug resistance.
4. Underutilization of contraceptive pills may cause pregnancy.

Overutilization of Drugs

It means more or extra consumption of drugs than prescribed.

Consumption of OTC drugs, consumption of drug when it is not needed, consumption of same medication from different containers, consumption of number of doses more than prescribed, are the causes of overutilization.

Consequences of overutilization depends upon type of drug, type of disease, type of patient and quantity of drug, e.g.

1. Overutilization of tobacco and alcohol can cause their addiction.
2. Overutilization of caffeine causes psychological dependence.
3. Overutilization of antacid causes constipation.
4. Overutilization of sodium chloride can cause hypertension.

6 Write about 'medication history of the patient'. (S. 09; W. 01)

☞ Medication History

"It is the collective information of the patient about his body disorders, drug allergies and other information."

It is the job of the pharmacist to take the complete medication history of the patient.

Medication history provides vital information about the patient.

Objectives of Taking Medication History

1. To develop a list of the patient's current and past medications.
2. To determine if the patient has allergies or adverse reactions with some drugs.
3. To know about patients self-prescribing habits or to study the tendency of OTC drugs.
4. To study the ability of the patient to show compliance.
5. To maintain essential information of the patient.
6. To study refilling frequency of patient.
7. To know about habits of the patient.
8. For adjustment of better drug therapy.

9. To avoid drug-drug interaction.
10. To reduce overutilization of drugs.

Medication history includes information about:

1. Name
2. Age
3. Sex
4. Date of birth
5. Address, phone, fax
6. Family background
7. Economical and social status
8. Tendency about the consumption of medicines
9. Views and way of thinking of patients
10. Habits
11. Body disorders
12. Drug allergies
13. Tendency of taking OTC drugs
14. Previous diseases
15. Previous medicines consumed, etc.

Method of Taking Medication History

1. The medication history should be collected and maintained by clinical pharmacist.
2. It is collected by asking some direct and indirect questions.
3. It should be completed within 24 to 40 hours after his hospitalisation.
4. Clinical pharmacist should provide minimum privacy and confidence to the patient.
5. He should ask some time efficient questions.

General Format of Medication History

Medication History

Name: Age: Sex: Birth date:

Address: Phone No:

Family background: Previous diseases:

Drug allergies: Drugs used:

Body disorder: Prescriber's name:

Adverse effects suffered: Non-prescribed drugs:

Consumption of: Yes/No

(i) Caffeine
(ii) Alcohol
(iii) Tobacco
(iv) Morphine, heroin

Importance of Medication History

1. It gives vital information about patient compliance.
2. To avoid probable allergic hypersensitivity reactions.
3. To cousel the patient.
4. To adjust better drug therapy to the patient.

7 What advice must be given to the patient using following drugs (important for all examinations)?

☞

Drugs	Advice
1. Salicylate (aspirin)	Do not take on empty stomach.
2. Antacid tablet	Not to be swallowed, to be chewed.
3. MAO inhibitors	Avoid eating of cheese, chocolate and alcoholic beverages.
4. Tetracyclines	Do not take with milk or with antacids.
5. Phenobarbitone or phenytoin	Expose yourself to sunlight in the morning.
6. Diazepam	(i) Do not drink alcohol. (ii) Do not work on dangerous machinery. (iii) Do not use for prolonged time. (iv) Do not drive a vehicle.
7. Antiepileptics	Avoid alcohol consumption.
8. Phenolphthalein	It may colour urine and stool to pink.
9. Liquid paraffin	Do not use for prolonged time.
10. Metronidazole	Avoid alcohol consumption.
11. Caffeine	It is mild habit forming.
12. Boric acid	Contraindicated in children below 12 years old.
13. Vaginal contraceptives (chemical contraceptives)	(i) Insert about 10 minutes before intercourse. (ii) Each suppository remains effective only for 1 hour.
14. Diphenhydramine	It may cause sedation.
15. Phenylbutazone, oxyphenbutazone	Do not take on empty stomach.
16. Spermicidal jellies or creams	Creams and gellies should be applied for 10 to 20 min before

Contd.

Drugs	Advice
	intercourse and these are effective and should remain in vagina for 6 to 8 hr.
17. Ampicillin	(i) It should be taken on empty stomach, i.e. at least 1 hr before or 2 hr after food consumption. (ii) It may cause diarrhoea if it is severe, consult the physician. (iii) Do not stop its administration earlier than recommended by doctor even if you may feel better otherwise infection may reoccur.
18. Emulsion and suspensions	Shake well before use.
19. Oral pills	Should be taken regularly.
20. Eyedrops	(i) How to remove the seal and how to instill in eye should be demonstrated. (ii) Do not touch the tip of a dropper. (iii) Use the solution within 1 month.
21. Antibiotics	Take complete prescribed course.
22. Antidiabetics	Avoid alcoholic beverages.
23. Sulpha drugs	Take a large amount of fluid and alkali or water.
24. Chloramphenicol	(i) Frequent blood count taken during prolonged administration. (ii) Avoid prolonged therapy.
25. Haematinics	It may colour the faeces reddish brown.
26. Aluminium hydroxide	Constipation may occur.

11

Medical Terminology

1 Explain the terms. Give meaning of following medical terms.

1. Amoebiasis: Amoebiasis is an infectious disease caused by protozoa, *Entamoeba histolytica*.
2. Anaesthetic: It means a substance which reduces pains by making the individual unconscious.
3. Counter irritants: It means the drugs that counteract irritation and thereby relieving pains.
4. Laxatives: The drugs which promote defaecation.
5. Immunity: It means the power of body to resist infection.
6. Emetics: The drugs which induce vomiting are called emetics.
7. Analeptics: The drugs which stimulate CNS are called analeptics.
8. Cholagogue: The drugs which increase secretion of bile.
9. Sialogogue: The drugs which increase secretion of saliva.
10. Galactogogue: The drugs which increase secretion of milk.
11. Hydrogogue: The drug which produces fluid motions.
12. Tranquillizers: The drugs which produce calming and quietening effect on the minds of patients are called tranquillizers.
13. Astringents: The drugs which cause precipitation of superficial proteins of the skin.
14. Acidosis: It means increased acid reserve in the body.
15. Alkalosis: It means increased alkali reserve in the body.
16. Hyperuricaemia: Increased level of uric acid in blood.

17. Hypokalaemia: Low level of potassium in blood.
18. Oliguria: Less urine formation.
19. Anaemia: Decrease in number of RBCs.
20. Polycythaemia: Increase in number of RBCs.
21. Leukaemia: Increase in number of WBCs.
22. Leucopaenia: Decrease in number of WBCs.
23. Aplastic anaemia: Defective formation of RBC.
24. Blood dyscrasis: An abnormality of blood cells.
25. Agranulocytosis: Marked reduction in granulocyte count.
26. Haemolysis: Destruction of RBCs.
27. Thrombocytopaenia: Marked decrease in platelet count.
28. Actinomycosis: It is a fungal disease caused by actinomyces.
29. Arthritis: Inflammation of joints.
30. Carcinoma: Cancer.
31. Congenital: Existing from birth.
32. Diaphoresis: Sweating, perspiration.
33. Embolism: Obstruction of blood flow due to clot, air or tumour cells.
34. Enuresis: Bed wetting.
35. Iatrogenic: Drug-induced diseases.
36. Ischaemia: Condition due to reduced blood supply.
37. Aetiology: Cause of disease.
38. Parturition: Act of bearing a child.
39. Postpartum: After birth.
40. Rhinitis: Swelling of nasal mucous membrane.
41. Spasm: A sudden, violent involuntary contraction of muscle.
42. Teratogen: A substance which can cause foetal abnormality.
43. Tumour: A mass of abnormal tissue growth due to cancer.
44. Virilism: Presence of male characters in females.
45. Amnesia: Loss of memory.
46. Analgesia: Loss of pain sensation.
47. Anxiety: A feeling of uneasiness, tension.
48. Delirium: Abnormal mental condition.
49. Dizziness: A sensation of falling.
50. Coma: Deep sleep with complete loss of consciousness.
51. Epilepsy: A disease of brain due to abnormal electrical discharge.
52. Euphoria: A feeling of well being.
53. Hallucination: A sensation of false perception without sensory stimulus.

54. Lethargy: Sluggishness.
55. Mania: A mental depressive disease.
56. Meningitis: Inflammation of meninges due to infection.
57. Motion sickness: A feeling of nausea and vomiting during travelling.
58. Migraine: A severe sudden headache.
59. Narcosis: Drug-induced unconsciousness.
60. Ototoxic: Toxicity in ear.
61. Parasthesia: Abnormality of sensation.
62. Parkinsonism: A degenerative syndrome of CNS due to cholinergic dopaminergic imbalance.
63. Peripheral neuritis: Inflammation of peripheral nerves.
64. Stupor: Loss of consciousness.
65. Tinitus: A ringing sound in ear.
66. Trauma: Due to external force, a wound or injury is produced.
67. Tremor: Involuntary muscular movements.
68. Vertigo: A sensation of rotation of oneself.
69. Insomnia: It means lack of sleep.
70. Miosis: Constriction of pupil.
71. Mydriatic: Dilatation of pupil.
72. Cycloplegia: Paralysis of ciliary muscles of eye leading to loss of accommodation.
73. Conjunctivitis: Inflammation of conjunctiva.
74. Diplopia: Double vision.
75. Iritis: Inflammation of iris.
76. Night blindness: Absence of vision in dark due to deficiency of vitamin A
77. Glaucoma: Increased intra-ocular tension.
78. Photophobia: Difficulty to expose eyes to light
79. Acnes: A common skin disease
80. Alopecia: Loss of hair leading to baldness.
81. Anaphylaxis: A severe hypersensitivity.
82. Cyanosis: A bluish tinge observed under nails, lips and skin due to lack of oxygenated haemoglobin.
83. Erythema: Reddening of skin.
84. Pruritis: Itching.
85. Inflammation: A reaction of tissue to injury.
86. Apnoea: Temporary cessation of respiration.
87. Dyspnoea: Difficulty in breathing.

88. Hypoxia: Deficiency of O_2 in tissues.
89. Anoxia: Lack of O_2 in tissues.
90. Demulscent: An agent producing soothing and protective action.
91. Arrhythmia: Abnormal rhythm of heart.
92. Bradycardia: Decrease in heart rate.
93. Tachycardia: Increase in heart rate.
94. Angina: Pains in the chest due to less O_2 supply to myocardium.
95. Myocardial infarction: Damage to myocardium due to inadequate blood supply.
96. Ionotrophy: It means force of contraction of heart.
97. Chronotrophy: It means rate of heart.
98. Anorexia: Loss of appetite.
99. Colitis: Swelling of colon.
100. Dyspepsia: Indigestion.
101. Dysphagia: Difficulty in swallowing (deglutition).
102. Glossitis: Inflammatory tongue.
103. Heart burn: Due to hyperacidity, gastric contents come into mouth causing a burning sensation in chest.
104. Paralytic ileus: Paralysis of intestinal muscles.
105. Achlorhydria: Absence of hydrochloric acid secretion by gastric gland.
106. Diarrhoea: Excretion of watery stools.
107. Libido: Desire of sex.
108. Menopause: Menstrual cycle termination.
109. Neonates: Newborn up to 1 month.
110. Infant: Child less than 1 year old.
111. Micturition: Act of urination.
112. Dysmenorrhoea: Painful menstruation.
113. Medicine: It is the term explaining all the aspects of sciences of prevention, investigation and treatment of diseases.
114. Disease: It means some abnormality in structure or function of body.
115. Acute: It means rapid onset and rapid progress.
116. Chronic: It means slow onset and slow progress.
117. Organic: Associated with abnormality in structure or organ.
118. Acquired: Acquired after birth.
119. Congenital: Present at birth.
120. Familial: Occurring in families.

121. Systemic: Involving in body system.
122. Local: Involving only a part of body.
123. Neoplastic: Formation of tumour.
124. Infective: Due to infection.
125. Allergy: Due to hypersensitivity.
126. Psychiatric: Due to abnormality in mind.
127. Semiparalysis: Paralysis of one side of body.
128. Paraplegia: Paralysis of legs.
129. Saluresis: Excretion of sodium and chloride ions in urine.
130. Pathogenesis: It refers to development of diseases.

2 Translate the Latin terms into English.

☞ 1. Tussis: Cough
2. Secundus: Every two
3. Gutta: Drop
4. Libra: Pound
5. Die: Day
6. Cataplasma: Poultice
7. Semel: Once
8. Ter: Thrice
9. Succus: Juice
10. Unus: One
11. Ante cibos: Before meals
12. Post cibos: After meals
13. Hora: An hour
14. Pulvis: A powder
15. Statim: Immediately
16. Duo: Two
17. Decem: Ten
18. Ut ditum: As directed
19. Quarter: Four time
20. Semis: One half

3 Explain the following terms in brief.

☞ 1. **Brand name:** It is the trade name of the drug. This name is privately owned by the manufacturer or distributor, e.g. paracetamol tab brand name: Crocin.

2. **Generic names:** These are the official, common or public names used to designate an active drug entity, whether in pure form or in dosage form.
    - Many drugs are marketed under the generic names of the principle active ingredient and do not bear brand names of the manufacturer.
    - Generic compounds are listed in schedule 'W' of D & C Act 1940, e.g. paracetamol, ampicillin, chlorpromazine, etc.
3. **Over-the-counter drugs/OTC drug:** These are the drug products that can be purchased without prescription. Because of the unrestricted availability of these drugs many people do consider OTC medicines as drugs.
4. **Polypharmacy:** It refers to the concurrent use of many drugs during the course of treatment for a particular illness.
5. **Contraindication:** It is the condition where the drugs should not be given, e.g. penicillin should not be given to allergic patients.
6. **Super infection:** It means development of secondary infection during the course of primary infection.

12

Pathophysiology and Symptoms of Diseases

1 Explain the terms aetiology, pathogenesis and lesion. (S. 96)

☞ • **Aetiology:** Aetiology means actual cause of a disease.
- **Pathogenesis:** It means development or evolution of diseases.
- **Lesion:** A demonstrable structural change produced in the course of a disease is referred to as lesion.

2 Write the manifestations and pathophysiology of 'tuberculosis'. (S. 96, 97, 98, 02, 04, 07, 08; W. 98, 99, 01, 03, 08)

☞ Tuberculosis is a bacterial infection caused by *Mycobacterium tuberculosis*.

Pathophysiology

Tubercle bacilli are inhaled through respiratory system and are deposited in peripheral alveoli throughout lungs. Then the bacilli are drained to lymph nodes and circulated throughout the body through bloodstream.

Types of Tuberculosis

(a) Primary tuberculosis
(b) Pulmonary tuberculosis
(c) Miliary tuberculosis.

Manifestations, Signs and Symptoms

1. Coughing
2. Fatigue
3. Weight loss
4. Cough early in the morning, green or yellow sputum with blood
5. Dyspnoea
6. Weakness
7. Fever
8. Night sweats
9. GIT disturbances
10. Ulceration of bronchial mucosa.

Drugs used to Control/Treat TB

1. Isoniazid
2. Rifampicin
3. Ethambutol
4. Pyrazinamide
5. Streptomycin
6. PAS
7. Cycloserine
8. Thiacetazone

3 Write the manifestations and pathophysiology of diabetes. (S. 98, 99, 00, 01, 02, 07, 09; W. 03, 05, 08)

☞ Diabetes mellitus is a chronic disease characterized by a state of chronic hyperglycaemia and is caused due to deficiency of insulin.

Aetiology: It may be caused due to some viral infections damaging cells of Langerhans which causes insulin deficiency.

Pathophysiology: Lower levels of insulin result in over production of hepatic glucose and its underutilization. This results in hyperglycaemia. Hyperglycaemia results in glycosuria.

Types of Diabetes

Depending upon the insulin levels diabetes in divided into two categories.

1. Insulin-dependant or juvenile diabetes.
2. Insulin non-dependant or maturity onset diabetes.

Signs and Symptoms (Manifestations)

1. Hyperglycaemia
2. Glycosuria
3. Polyuria
4. Polydypsia
5. Weight loss
6. Dehydration
7. Decreased muscle strength
8. Bed wetting

9. Oliguria
10. Hypotension
11. Retinopathy
12. Ketoacidosis

Treatments

Drugs

1. Insulin
2. Chlorpropamide
3. Tolbutamide
4. Glibenclamide
5. Phenformin
6. Metformin

4 Write the manifestations and pathophysiology of epilepsy. (S. 05)

☞ Epilepsy

It is a chronic disorder of cerebral functions characterized by repeated sudden attacks of seizures usually lasting for about 10 minutes.

Aetiology: Brain tumours, accidental CNS damages, infections, etc. may cause seizures.

Pathophysiology: Normally electric charges are generated by neuronal cells which are called neuronal discharges in response to a stimulus. These discharges are carried to neighbouring neuronal cells and axons. Sudden excessive, discharges lead to convulsions.

Types of Epilepsy

1. Grandmal epilepsy
2. Petitmal epilepsy
3. Motor epilepsy
4. Focal cortical epilepsy
5. Minor epilepsy.

Signs and Symptoms (Manifestations)

1. Generalized convulsions
2. Sudden loss of consciousness
3. A crying
4. Falling
5. Clonic movements of muscles
6. Loss of control over various activities
7. Eyelid blinking.

Drug Treatment

1. Phenytoin
2. Methoin
3. Ethosuximide
4. Carbamazepine
5. Phenobarbitone
6. Primidone

5 Give manifestations and pathophysiology of peptic ulcer. (S. 99; W. 00, 02, 06)

☞ Peptic Ulcer

Peptic ulcer disease includes ulceration anywhere in the GIT where parietal cells secrete hydrochloric acid.

Types of Peptic Ulcers

1. Duodenal ulcer

It is a peptic ulcer in the wall of the duodenum.

Pathophysiology

1. It is related to excessive secretion of HCl by the parietal cells in the stomach.
2. Half the patients with duodenal ulcer show gastric hyper-secretion. It is due to increased parietal cell mass, excessive gastrin release during meal, high sensitivity to gastrin.
3. It occurs more frequently in patients with hyperthyroidisms, alcoholic cirrhosis and rheumatoid arthritis.

Signs and Symptoms

1. Inflammation of duodenal mucosa
2. Burning pains
3. Weight loss
4. Patient may show iron deficiency anaemia.

2. Gastric ulcer

It is the ulcer in stomach. It is more common in men than women and usually occurs after fifty years of age.

Pathophysiology

1. Gastric ulcer is primarily due to the breakdown of mucosal barrier.
2. Cigarette smoking and ingestion of salicylates increase the risk of developing gastric ulcer.

Signs and Symptoms

1. Gastric pain which is reduced by food.
2. The pain in gastric ulcer is burning but less localized than the duodenal ulcers.
3. Gastric ulcer pain generally does not occur at night.

Drug Treatment

1. Aluminium hydroxide gel
2. Magnesium hydroxide
3. Cimetidine
4. Ranitidine.

6 Give the manifestations and pathophysiology of hepatitis. (W. 98)

☞ Hepatitis

- Hepatitis is an inflammation of the liver. Causes of hepatitis include viral and bacterial infections, autoimmune disorders and exposure to chemicals.
- There are four types of viruses causing different types of hepatitis.

Hepatitis A virus	→	Hepatitis A
Hepatitis B virus	→	Hepatitis B
Delta virus	→	Delta hepatitis.
		Hepatitis non-A and non-B

- Hepatitis A virus is an RNA virus usually contracted by oral-faecal exposure to an infected individual.
- Hepatitis B virus is a DNA virus generally acquired by parenteral exposure to contaminated blood products or infected syringes.

Pathophysiology

The hepatitis B virus replicates in the liver cells and virus cells and gets incorporated in the liver cell membranes. Thus, it damages the liver.

Mode of Transmission

1. Faecal or oral route
2. Parenteral route
3. Sexual transmission

Signs and Symptoms

1. Anorexia
2. Fatigue
3. Vomiting, nausea
4. Headache
5. Photophobia
6. Changes in sense of smell and taste
7. Chills, fever
8. Pharyngitis and cough
9. Epigastric discomfort
10. Urine darkens and stools get coloured.

7 Name various CVS disorders. Write pathophysiology and manifestations of hypertension. (W. 03)

☞ CVS Disorders

A. Disorders of Heart

1. Congenital heart disease
2. Congestive heart failure (CHF)
3. Coronary heart disease (CHD)
4. Ischemic heart disease (IHD)
5. Angina pectoris
6. Cardiac arrhythmia
7. Heart block
8. Hypertension
9. Hypotension
10. Rheumatic heart disease.

B. Disorders of Blood Vessels

Disorders of Arteries

1. Arteriosclerosis
2. Arteritis.

Disorders of veins: Varicosed vein.

Hypertension (W. 98)

An abnormal increase in blood pressure is called hypertension. Hypertension is often defined as the increase in systolic pressure above 150 mmHg and diastolic above 90 mmHg.

Types of Hypertension

1. Primary hypertension
2. Secondary hypertension.

Pathophysiology

Hypertension itself is a risk factor for arteriosclerosis and CVS complications like angina pectoris, CHF. Chronic hypertension results in damage to end organs like eyes, brain, kidney and heart.

Signs and Symptoms

1. Retinopathy: Blurred vision leading to blindness.
2. CNS symptoms: Lethargy, confusion, convulsions and coma.
3. CVS disorders like angina pectoris or CCF.
4. Deposition of fibrin in glomerulus.

Drug Treatment

1. Methyl dopa
2. Clonidine
3. Reserpine
4. Guanethidine
5. Mecamylamine.

13

Physiological Parameters

1 Define physiological parameters. Give the normal values and significance of them. (S. 98, 00; W. 00, 02)

☞ Definition

Physiological parameters are nothing but normal values for various body fluids and their composition, normal functioning rates of organs which helps in the diagnosis of diseases and disorders.

Parameter	Normal range	Significance/Importance
1. Haemoglobin	Male: 15.5 ± 2.5 gm% Female: 14 ± 2.5 gm% Infants: Up to 18 gm%	↓sed in anaemia ↑sed in polycythaemia, dehydration
2. RBC count-(Erythrocytes)	Male: 4.5 to 5.5 million/mm^3 Female: 3.5 to 5.5 million/mm^3 Children 4 to 5.5 million/mm^3	↓sed in anaemia, pregnancy old age ↑sed in polycythaemia, cholera, burns, chronic heart disease.
3. WBC count (Leucocytes) (TLC) (Total leucocyte count)	4000 to 11,000 / mm^3	↓sed in leucopenia, influenza, typhoid, hepatitis, agranulocytosis. ↑sed in leukaemia pneumonia, tonsilitis, meningitis, appedicitis.
4. Differential leucocyte count (DLC)	Neutrophils: 60 to 70% Eosinophils: 1 to 4 %	↑sed in pneumonia, tonsilitis ↑sed in allergic conditions, skin diseases.

Contd.

Parameter	Normal range	Significance/Importance
	Basophils: 0 to 1%	↑sed in granulocytic leukaemia.
	Monocytes: 5 to 10%	↑sed in malaria, typhoid, leukaemia, TB
	Lymphocytes: 25 to 30%	↑sed in whooping cough, typhoid, leukaemia, viral infection.
5. Platelet count (Thrombocytes)	3 to 4 lakhs	↓sed in thrombocytopenia (purpura)
6. Bleeding time	1 to 3 min (Dukes method)	↑sed in haemophilia.
7. Clotting time	2 to 6 minute by capillary method	↑sed in deficiency of vit.K, jaundice, pneumonia.
8. ESR (Erythrocyte sedimentation rate)	Method — M — F (i) Western Green — 0–15 — 0–20 (ii) Cutler — 0–8 — 0–10 (iii) Wintrobe — 0–9 — 0–15	ESR is ↑sed in rheumatic fever, rheumatoid arthritis, nephritis TB, leukaemia, metallic poisoning.
9. Prothrombin time	10–14 sec	Prolonged in liver diseases.
10. Thrombin time	20–29 sec	Prolonged in liver diseases.
11. Heart rate/ beats	Males: 65 to 70 Females: 70 to 80	↑sed in emotional excitement, fever, muscular exercise.
12. Blood pressure	120/80 mmHg.	↑sed BP causes hypertension ↓sed BP cause hypotension.
13. Mean corpuscular volume (MCV)	Adult: 80–96	↓sed in anaemia
14. Mean cell Hb conc. (MCHC)	32–36%	↓sed in anaemia.
15. Blood sugar	80–120 mg/100 ml	↑sed in diabetes, anaesthesia ↓sed in pancreatic tumour, insulin overdose.
16. Cholesterol	In adult: 150–240 mg%	↑sed in nephrosis, diabetes arteriosclerosis ↓sed in hyperthyroidism myxoedema.
17. Sperm count	60–150 million/cc	Below normal range may indicate infertility

Contd.

Parameter	Normal range	Significance/Importance
18. Cerebrospinal Fluid Examination (CSF)		
(a) Appearance	: Clear, colourless, does not clot on standing.	
(b) Colour	: (Abnormal)	
(c) Turbidity	: (Abnormal)	
(d) Coagulate	: (Abnormal)	
(e) RBCs	: Nil	
(f) Proteins	: Low (15–40 mg/100 ml)	
(g) Glucose	: 40 to 70 mg/100 ml in adult	
(h) Chloride	: 650–750 mg NaCl/100 ml	

Significance of CSF Examination

		Significance
(a) Colour	- Presence of blood	In tumour, haemorrhage
(b) Turbidity	- Presence of cells or organisms	In meningitis.
(c) Coagulate	- Presence of fibrinogen	In TB, spinal tumour
(d) Proteins	- Increased	In inflammation, brain and spinal tumour
(e) Glucose	- Decreased	In meningitis
	- Increased	In brain tumours, diabetes
(f) Chloride	- Decreased	In meningitis

19. Urine Examination

Parameter	Normal range	Significance/Importance
1. Volume	1200–2000 ml/day	↑sed urine output called polyuria. No urine output then anuria.
2. Specific gravity	1.005– 1.025	↑ sed in diabetes ↓ sed in chronic nephritis.
3. pH	4.8 to 7.5	↓sed pH below 4.8 in diabetes.
4. Epithelial cells	Traces in normal urine	↑sed in nephritis.
5. Casts (Degenerative tissues)	Traces in normal urine	↑sed in renal irritation
6. RBCs	–	Tumour of bladder or kidney, nephritis
7. Crystals	Appear when stands for long	
8. Abnormal constituents		
(a) Proteins	Proteinuria	In nephritis, renal TB, pregnancy
(b) Sugar	Glycosuria	In diabetes mellitus.
(c) Ketone bodies	Ketonuria	In carbohydrate starvation, anaesthesia.
(d) Bile salts	–	In jaundice
(e) Blood cells	Haematuria	In TB cancer, kidney stones haemolysis, poisoning.
(f) Pus cells	Pyuria	Nephritis, kidney lesions

Contd.

Parameter	Normal range	Significance/Importance
20. Stool Examination		
1. Consistency	Semisolid	Infection shows watery stools
2. Colour	Brownish	Change in colour, diet, drugs and internal bleeding
3. Odour (smell)	Specific	A very foul smell indicates ulceration, lesions in lower colon, rectum.
4. Mucus	Small amount	Large amount in dysentery, amoebiasis, colitis.
5. Cells	–	Observed in amoebic and bacillary dysentery.
6. Common parasites	–	Observed in presence of hookworm threadworm infestation.

SURGICAL INSTRUMENTS, HOSPITAL EQUIPMENTS AND HEALTH ACCESSORIES

2 Define "surgical instruments". Enlist different surgical equipments along with their types and uses. (S. 96, 97, 98, 02, 03, 04, 09; W. 98, 00, 05)

☞ Surgical Instruments

The instruments which are commonly used in surgical operations are called surgical instruments.

(A) Scissors (W. 96)

Scissors are the metal instruments mainly used to cut the tissues or muscles.

1. Straight blunt scissors
2. Straight pointed scissors
3. Angled scissors (pointed or blunt)
4. Stitch cutting scissors
5. Lister's bandage scissors to cut the bandage.

(B) Forceps

Forceps are the surgical instruments used to hold the tissues during separation of tissues or preventing blood flow.

1. **Tissue forceps:** These are used to hold the tissues.
   (a) Toothed tissue forceps:

(i) Allis type
(ii) Lane's type
(iii) Moynihans type

(b) Non-toothed tissue forceps, e.g. Bobcock's tissue forceps.

2. **Haemostatic or artery forceps:** These are used to prevent blood flow.
3. **Dissecting forceps:** These are used to facilitate clear operative field.
4. **Bone-cutting forceps:** These are used to cut bone. They have a sharp blade and handle with or without lever system.
5. **Forceps used to hold and pick up surgical accessories:**
   (i) Grays towel clip
   (ii) Doyens type
6. Tongue-holding forceps.
7. Sponge-holding forceps
8. **Piles holding forceps:** These are used to hold pile mass.

(C) Needles and Needle Holders

(i) **Needles used for suturing**: These are used for sewing the tissue together with stitches, e.g. straight needle, round shaft curved needle, flat shaft curved needle, lumbar puncture needle and anerysm needle.

(ii) **Hypodermic needles:** These are attached with syringes and available in various sizes, e.g.

Parenteral needles: (i) Reusable (steel)
(ii) Dispoable

(iii) **Needle holder:** It is used to hold needles during saturing, so the chances of contaminations are reduced.

(D) Catheters (S. 03)

These are rubber tubings which are inserted in some organs directly through natural openings.

1. **Simple rubber catheter:** They are used to drain urine.
2. **Self-retaining Foley's balloon catheter:** They are used to drain urine.
3. **Rectal catheters or tubes:** These are used to remove faeces or gases from return.

4. **Stomach tube:** For aspiration of the stomach contents and for feeding.
5. **Oxygen, sterile tubes:** For extension and connection of air passages to provide oxygenation.
6. **Nasal catheters:** For introduction of inhalants in asthma cases and to induce general anaesthesia.

3 Name various equipment/machineries used in hospitals along with their diagnostic uses/significance.

☞ Hospital Equipment

1. **ECG machine:** To record electrocardiogram and to study working of heart.
2. **Sphygmomanometer:** It is used to measure blood pressure.
3. **X-ray machine:** It is used to take internal photographs of body and helps in diagnosis of disorders.
4. **Ultrasound sonography:** This equipment records images of internal abdominal organs and is used as a diagnostic tool. It is generally used in gynaecologic and obstetrics practice.
5. **Doppler echocardiography:** It is an ultrasound recording device used to diagnose heart diseases.
6. **Lithotripsy:** It is a non-invasive technique used to break up urinary stones by a laser beam.
7. **Glucometer:** It is used to estimate blood glucose level in a minute.
8. **CT scanner:** They are highly developed, computerized machines which record morphology of internal soft organs. They are used for diagnostic purpose where X-ray machines are not enough.
9. **Magnetic Image Resonance (MIR):** It is a highly modernized diagnostic tool in complicated cases.

4 What do you mean by health accessories? Enlist any three with their uses.

☞ Health Accessories

Health accessories are specially prepared equipments which are used to reduce disability. Health accessories should be selected according to age, lifestyle, disability-related factors.

Examples:

(i) **Wheelchairs:** These are the chairs having wheels at the base. These chairs are useful for mobility of the patients disabled in lower extremities (legs).

(ii) **Walkers:** This accessory gives support to the patient while walking.

(iii) **Hospital beds:** They may be manual or electrically operated.

14

Drug Interactions

1 Define and classify various types of drug interactions. (S. 96, 97, 98, 00, 07; W. 02, 04, 05)

☞ Definition

Drug interactions are defined as the alteration in pharmacological response of the drug due to presence of other substance or drug.

Or

Drug interaction is an alteration of effect of one drug by prior or concurrent administration of another drug.

Classification

According to mechanism drug interactions are classified as follows:

Drug interactions

A. Pharmaceutical drug interactions	B. Pharmacokinetic drug interactions	C. Pharmacodynamic drug interactions
(a) Chemical (b) Physical	(a) Alteration in absorption (b) Alteration in distribution (c) Alteration in metabolism (d) Alteration in excretion	(a) Due to opposite pharmacological effect. (b) Due to similar pharmacological effect (c) Alteration of electrolyte levels. (d) Alteration at receptor sites (e) Interaction with formulating additives.

2 Give the significance/importance of drug interactions.

☞ Significance/Importance of Drug Interactions

1. To produce synergistic effect.
2. To get an important therapeutic effect.
3. To provide greater margin of safety.
4. To get a more appropriate onset of duration of action.
5. To lower toxicity of drugs.
6. To enhance or increase the potency of drug.
7. Highly improved therapy is possible by use of drug interactions.
8. To modify effects of drug by prior administration, e.g. preanaesthetic medication.

3 Describe various pharmacokinetic drug interactions. (S. 97, 00, 02, 04; W. 01, 08)

☞ Pharmacokinetic Drug Interactions

In this type, absorption, distribution, metabolism and excretion of drug can be modified by other agents.

1. Alteration in Absorption

Alteration in absorption may be due to following factors:

(i) Alteration in pH
(ii) Inhibition of GIT enzymes
(iii) Change in osmotic pressure
(iv) Adsorption
(v) Complextion
(vi) Food

For example,

(i) Antacids decrease absorption of acidic drugs and increase absorption of basic drugs.
(ii) Kaolin adsorbs tetracycline and digoxin-like drugs therefore, their absorption is decreased.
(iii) Purgatives increase gastric motility therefore, absorption of digoxin-like drug is decreased.
(iv) Atropine decreases motility of GIT therefore, absorption of some drugs is late but sustained action is obtained.

(v) Antimicrobials change microbial flora of GIT therefore, absorption of vitamins is decreased and also anticoagulant effect of anticoagulants.

(vi) Phenytoin inhibits intestinal enzymes therefore, absorption of folic acid is increased.

2. Alteration in Distribution of Drugs

Alteration in distribution of drug may be due to change in drug transport or due to protein binding of drugs.

For example,

(i) Salicylates break binding of tolbutamide from their binding site thus cause severe hypoglycemia.

(ii) Phenylbutazone replaces warfarin from protein binding therefore, warfarin serum level is increased thus prolongs anticoagulant effect.

3. Alteration in Metabolism of Drug

Alterations in metabolism are due to enzyme inhibition or increase in metabolism.

For example,

(i) Barbiturates stimulate metabolic degradation of alcohol and phenytoin due to stimulation of liver enzyme therefore, their effects are reduced.

(ii) Phenylbutazone inhibits metabolism of tolbutamide therefore, prolongs hypoglycemic effect.

4. Alterations in Excretion of Drugs

Alterations in excretion of drugs may be due to:

(i) Inhibition of excretion

(ii) Change in urinary pH

(iii) Increase in renal excretion

(iv) Change in tubular transport system.

For example,

(i) Quinidine decreases excretion of digoxin. Thus toxicity of digoxin occurs.

(ii) Sodium bicarbonate increases excretion of salicylates and barbiturates. Thus, it is useful in treatment of salicylate and barbiturate poisoning.

(iii) Acidic drugs are rapidly excreted in basic urine.

(iv) Antacids make urine alkaline therefore, ionization of salicylates and barbiturate occurs which further causes rapid excretion of these drugs.

(v) Probencid decreases excretion of penicillin.

4 Describe pharmacodynamic drug interactions. (S. 98, 03, 05, 06, 09; W. 06)

☞ Pharmacodynamic Drug Interactions

Pharmacodynamic interactions are beneficial or harmful.

1. **Due to opposite pharmacological effect:** If two drugs are administered which are having opposite effect, i.e. one drug blocks the action of another drug and leads to drug interaction, e.g.
   (i) Atropine blocks the actions of pilocarpine,
   (ii) Alcohol and amphetamine shows opposite effects on CNS.
2. **Due to similar pharmacological effect:** If two drugs and administered having similar effect, it may produce synergistic effect, e.g.
   (i) Sulphamethoxazole and trimethoprim both are bacteriostatic but their combination shows bacteriocidal effect.
   (ii) Toxicity of digitalis can be increased by thiazides.
   (iii) Aspirin and codeine produce good analgesic action.
3. Due to interaction with formulating additives, e.g. tetracycline with calcium.
4. **Alteration of electrolyte levels:** Some drugs cause alteration in fluid and electrolyte level balance, e.g. diuretics cause loss of potassium, may produce hypokalaemia in turn making heart more sensitive to digitalis.
5. **Drug interaction at receptor sites:** Effect of drugs occurs as a result of binding to specialised areas known as receptor sites.

5 Write a note on "drug-food interaction". (S. 99, 01; W. 96, 97, 06, 08)

☞ Drug-Food Interaction

It is an interaction due to concurrent administration of drug along with food materials.

Explanation

- Commonest route of administration of drug is oral or enteral. The presence of food in GIT affects bioavailability of drugs by changing absorption, distribution, metabolism and excretion of drug or by changing pharmacological action of drug.
- Drug-food interactions are either beneficial or harmful.
- Many times presence of food in GIT may change pharmacokinetic or dynamics of the drug.
- The drugs may be diluted due to presence of food and its absorption is delayed. This reduces risk of GIT irritation.

Examples

1. Metronidazole taken along with food causes nausea, vomiting, headache, can be avoided.
2. MAO inhibitors are contraindicated with tyramine containing foods (cheese, banana, chocolate, milk products) because MAO inhibitors inhibit MAO enzymes which is essential for metabolism of tyramine. Thus, level of tyramine increases and causes hypertensive crises, heart failure.
3. Tetracyclines form complexes with ions like calcium, magnesium, aluminium. Hence, milk or antacids should not be given along with tetracyclines.
4. Iron compounds are less absorbed in presence of food and in absence of food if iron is consumed causes nausea, vomiting. Therefore, iron preparation should be taken at least ½ an hour after consumption of food.
5. Acidic fruits cause decomposition of erythromycin and reduce its effect.
6. Egg, green vegetables decrease anticoagulant effect of warfarin because of increase in synthesis of vitamin K.

6 Elaborate different drug-drug interactions.

☞ Drug-Drug Interactions

A. Analgesic Drug Interactions

1. Salicylic acid	Ammoniated mercury	Skin irritation
2. Salicylates	Tolbutamide	Breaking of protein binding of tolbutamide causing "hypoglycaemia"

Contd.

3. Salicylates	Antacid (Sodium bicarbonate)	Rapid excretion of salicylate
4. Salicylate	Indomethacin	↑sed serum salicylate level
5. Aspirin	Heparin, warfarin	Anticoagulant activity increased.
6. Phenylbutazone	Warfarin, tolbutamide	Enhanced hypoglycaemic activity.
B. Diuretic Drug Interactions		
1. Thiazide	Quinidine	Quinidine serum level ↑sed
2. Thiazide	Tolbutamide, insulin	Thiazides antagonize effect of tolbutamide and insulin, therefore, dose of these drugs should be increased.
3. Thiazide	Alcohol	Alcohol increases hypotensive effect of thiazide thus causes severe hypertension.
4. Spironolactone	Potassium chloride	Hyperkalaemia
5. Thiazides	Digitalis glycosides	Hypokalaemia
6. Thiazide	Methyldopa, guanethidine	Excessive hypotension
7. Frusemide	Digitalis	Digitalis toxicity, renal toxicity.
C. Antidiabetic Drug Interactions (Hypoglycaemic)		
1. Tolbutamide	Thiazide	Thiazide antagonises effect of tolbutamide and, therefore, dose of hypoglycaemic agent should be increased.
2. Tolbutamide	Phenylbutazone	Increases hypoglycaemic activity
3. Tolbutamide	Salicylates	Increases hypoglycaemic activity
4. Tolbutamide	Sulphonamides	Sulpha drugs enhance hypoglycemic effect, therefore, dose should be adjusted.
5. Tolbutamide	Warfarin, heparin	↑ses hypoglycaemic activity
6. Tolbutamide	Oral contraceptives	Oral contraceptives develop glucose tolerance, i.e. oral contraceptives should not be used by diabetes patients.

Contd.

7. Phenformin metformin	Alcohol	Severe hypoglycaemia.

D. GIT Agents Drug Interactions

1. Sodium bicarbonate	Salicylates	Decrease GIT irritation
2. Potassium chloride	Spironolactone	Hyperkalaemia
3. Liquid paraffin	Anticoagulant	Due to decrease in absorption of vitamin K, effect of anticoagulant drug is increased.
4. Kaolin	Digoxin	Adsorbs digoxin. Thus decreases absorption of digoxin.
5. Sodium bicarbonate	Barbiturate	Increases excretion of barbiturate
6. Aluminium hydroxide gel	Isoniazid	↓ses absorption of isoniazid

E. Antihypertensive Drug Interactions

1. Guanethidine	MAO inhibitors	MAO inhibitors antagonise effect of guanethidine
2. Methyldopa	Ephedrine	Methyldopa reduces local mydriatic effect.
3. Methyldopa	Amphetamine	Amphetamine reduces hypotensive effect of methyldopa.
4. Reserpine	Atropine sulphate	Nasal decongestion due to reserpine blocked by atropine.
5. Reserpine	Ephedrine	Nasal decongestion due to reserpine, blocked by ephedrine.
6. Propranolol	MAO inhibitors	Severe hypertension occurs hence contraindicated.
7. Propranolol	Insulin	Propranolol binds blood sugar and also blocks clinical signs of hypoglycaemia. Therefore, ∴ Combination should be used with caution.

Contd.

F. Anticoagulant Drug Interactions

1. Warfarin, heparin	Tolbutamide	↑ses hypoglycaemic activity.
2. Warfarin, heparin	Aspirin	Increases anticoagulant activity
3. Anticoagulant	Liquid paraffin	Due to decrease in absorption of vitamin K, effect of anticoagulant is ↑sed.
4. Warfarin	Phenylbutazone	↑sed hypoglycaemic activity
5. Oral anticoagulant	Vitamin E	Anticoagulant effect is increased.
6. Heparin	Penicillin	Penicillin antagonises anticoagulant effect.
7. Warfarin, heparin	Streptomycin, sulphonamide, tetracycline, neomycin	These drugs increase anticoagulant effect.

G. Vitamin-Drug Interactions

1. Vitamin D	Phenytoin	Serum level of vitamin D is decreased.
2. Vitamin A	Mineral oil	Absorption of vitamin A is decreased.
3. Folic acid	Phenytoin	↓sed absorption of folic acid.
4. Vitamin B_6	Levodopa	↑sed metabolism of levodopa thus serum level is decreased.
5. Vitamin E	Oral anticoagulant	Anticoagulant effect is increased.
6. Pyridoxine	Barbiturate	↑ses metabolism of barbiturate
7. Pyridoxine	Oral contraceptive	↓ses level of pyridoxine
8. Vitamin C	Iron anticoagulant	↑ses absorption of iron ↓ses effect of anticoagulant.

H. Cardiovascular Drug Interactions

(a) Antiarrhythmic Drug Interactions

1. Procainamide	Sulphonamide	Antibacterial action is blocked.
2. Procainamide	Antihypertensives	More hypotensive effect
3. Procainamide	Cholinergic agents	Procainamide antagonises the effect of cholinergic drugs on skeletal muscle. Hence, should be avoided in myasthenic patients.

(b) Cardiac Glycoside Drug Interactions (Cardiotonic)

1. Digitalis	Thiazide	Hypokalaemia

Contd.

2. Digoxin	Kaolin	Adsorbs digoxin. Thus decreases absorption of digoxin
3. Digitalis glycosides	Phenylbutazone, barbiturates, phenytoin	These drugs enhance rate of metabolism of cardiac glycosides therefore, efficacy of cardiac glycosides decreases.

7 What are the reasons/causes of drug interactions?

☞ 1. **Administration of two or more drugs simultaneously:** In common practice more drugs are prescribed at a time which may be one of the main causes of drug interaction.
2. **Patient may refer many doctors/multi-prescription practice:** Sometimes patient is not satisfied by one doctor and may refer other doctors without informing about the previous consultation with the first doctor. This may result in taking the drugs which may interact with each other.
3. **Concurrent use of prescribed and non-prescribed drugs:** Patient may take the drugs like aspirin, paracetamol which are available without prescription. If such patients take other drugs prescribed by physician, drug interaction may occur and may be detrimental to the patient.
4. **Patient's non-compliance:** Sometimes patient does not comply with instructions given by physician, e.g. patient may take food which is being prohibited.
5. **Availability of potent drugs:** Potent drugs may interact with other drugs and thus may produce dangerous complications.

8 What is the role of pharmacist to avoid drug interactions?

☞ 1. Pharmacist should do patient counselling to make the patients aware about drug interactions.
2. Pharmacist should provide vital information about the drugs to patients regarding drug selection and administration.
3. Pharmacist working in hospitals should maintain drug history and medical record of the patient.
4. Pharmacist can educate the public for safe and effective use of medications through verbal communication as well as by written materials and use of computers.

15

Adverse Drug Reactions (ADRs)

1 Define and classify adverse drug reactions. (S. 97, 98, 99, 03, 05, 06, 07, 09; W. 96, 98, 00, 04, 05, 08)

☞ **Definition**

"It is defined as any undesirable, unintended response occurring at ordinary dose of drug, when drug is given for prophylaxis, diagnosis or treatment."

Classification of ADRs

- **A. Beneficial ADRs**
- **B. Harmful ADRs**
  - Predictable ADRs
    - (a) ADR due to excessive pharmacological action.
    - (b) ADR due to secondary pharmacological effect.
    - (c) ADR due to sudden withdrawal of drug.
  - Unpredictable ADRs
    - (a) Allergic reaction, e.g. skin rash, anaphylaxis.
    - (b) Genetically determined reactions.
    - (c) Idiosyncrasy.
    - (d) Teratogenicity.

2 What are the causes/reasons of adverse drug reactions? (S. 96, 05, 09; W. 97, 98, 02, 04, 08)

☞ (i) ADR due to improper prescription and dispensing: Sometimes improper doses are prescribed without taking patient's history.

(ii) Some drugs have very low margin of safety, i.e. therapeutic index.

(iii) Many formulations of different companies are therapeutically not equivalent due to difference in bioavailability and thus cause ADRs.

(iv) Some other factors such as presence of disease of liver or kidney may accumulate the drug in the body which can result in ADRs.

(v) Use of potent drugs also causes adverse drug reactions.

(vi) Genetic factor is also responsible for causing ADRs.

3 Write a note on "predictable adverse drug reactions". (W. 08)

☞ Definition

The adverse reactions whose cause is known or predictable are known as predictable ADRs.

These are usually related to pharmacological effects of drugs.

(a) Due to Excessive Pharmacological Action

- It is the most common ADR which may occur due to excessive pharmacological activity of drug.
- It is commonly seen with CNS depressants, hypoglycaemics, cardioactive agents and hypertensive agents.
- This type of reaction will develop in all patients, if excessive dosage is given.

  Examples:

  (i) Bradycardia is due to excessive effect of digoxin.

  (ii) Tetracyclines produce dermatitis.

  (iii) Clonidine produces rebound hypertension.

  (iv) Morphine produces severe bronchitis.

(b) Due to Secondary Pharmacological Effect

- There are very few drugs which produce a single pharmacological action, and most of the drugs produce more than one effect.
- The side effect may be sometimes adverse effects and such effects are called secondary pharmacological effects.

  Examples:

  (i) Patient receiving an antihistaminic for the prevention of motion sickness may become drowsy.

(ii) Antibiotics affect microflora of GIT therefore, absorption of vitamins is decreased. For this reason vitamins are supplemented with antibiotics.

(c) Due to Sudden Withdrawal of Drug

Chronic use of some drugs produces tolerance at cellular level and sudden withdrawal of such drugs produces severe adverse effects. Therefore, sudden withdrawal of drugs may show dangerous ADRs.

Examples:

(i) CNS depressants such as narcotics, barbiturates, alcohols, benzodiazepines show withdrawal symptoms such as confusion, delirium, prolonged depression and tachycardia.

(ii) Rebound hypertension is caused on sudden discontinuation of an antihypertensive agent, clonidine.

(iii) Sudden withdrawal of antiepileptic agents may cause rebound epileptic attacks.

4 Write a note on "unpredictable adverse drug reactions". (S. 00)

☞ Definition

Unpredictable ADRs are the unexpected responses produced by the drug due to repeated exposure of drug.

These are not known to the physician therefore, cannot be avoided or treated. These are not common with all patients.

Classification

(a) Allergic reactions, e.g. skin rash, anaphylaxis

(b) ADR due to genetic factor

(c) Idiosyncrasy

(d) Teratogenicity

(e) Iatrogenic disorders (doctor induced)

(a) **Allergy:** Allergy is an adverse response to a foreign substance resulting from a previous exposure to that substance.

- Allergy is also named as anaphylaxis or hypersensitivity reaction.

- The drugs showing allergic reactions are penicillins, sulpha drugs, quinine, tetracyclines, kanamycin, e.g.
  - (i) Penicillin causes difficulty in breathing, itching of skin, and decrease in BP.
  - (ii) Aspirin causes decrease in BP and haemolytic anaemia.
  - (iii) Methyldopa causes haemolytic anaemia.

(b) **ADR due to genetic factor:** These reactions are defined as genetically determined abnormal responses to a chemical. In this case these may be the inborn deficiency of certain enzyme systems to metabolism of particular drug therefore, shows allergic response to it, e.g. African people are having deficiency of glucose-phosphate dehydrogenase enzyme. Therefore, primaquine, dopsone, etc. cause acute haemolysis.

(c) **Idiosyncrasy (S. 96, 01, 05, 07)**

- When abnormal drug response occurs, the condition is called idiosyncrasy.
- It is a surprising ADR to physician.
- It is unusual individual response generally due to genetic variation.
- In addition, certain uncharacteristic drug effects due to peculiarities of an individual are included among idiosyncratic reactions.
- The term idiosyncrasy means
  - (i) idios means "one own"
  - (ii) synkrasis means "mixing together"

For example: (1) Thalidomide produces phocomelia
(2) Stilbesterol produces vaginal carcinoma.
(3) Analgesics may induce tumour of kidney pelvis in patients with renal disease.

(d) **Teratogenicity:** Teratogenicity is an ability of a drug to induce foetal abnormalities. The substances which cause such abnormalities of foetus development are called teratogens, e.g.

- (i) Thalidomide produces phocomelia.
- (ii) Stibesterol causes vaginal carcinoma.

(e) **Iatrogenic disorders (doctor induced):** These are the ADRs caused due to wrong prescription of drugs.

5 Define adverse drug reactions. Enlist factors affecting ADRs. What is the role of pharmacist in ADRs?

☞ **ADRs**

"It is defined as any undesirable, unintended response, occurring at ordinary dose of drug, when drug is given for prophylaxis, diagnosis or treatment."

Factors Affecting ADRs

1. Age
2. Sex
3. Tolerance
4. Genetic factor
5. Diet
6. Allergy
7. Environment
8. Type of drug therapy
9. Route of administration
10. Characteristic of drugs
11. Duration and multiple drug therapy

Role of Pharmacist in ADRs (W. 00, 01, 02, 04)

1. Pharmacist is an important link in between patients and physicians as he dispenses actual medicaments.
2. Pharmacist should give important information about the drugs to the patient regarding drug selection and administration.
3. Pharmacist should record the ADRs cases in hospital and should analyse them.
4. Pharmacist can educate the public for safe and effective use of medications through verbal communication as well as written materials, computers, etc.
5. Pharmacist is also expected to participate in post-marketing surveillance programs and to monitor for and prevent drug-induced diseases.
6. Pharmacist should study drug-drug, drug-diet and drug-disease interactions and time to time inform to the physicians, nurses and compounders, etc.
7. Pharmacist should do patient counselling so the possibilities of ADRs may be reduced.

6 Write a note on "teratogenicity". (S. 96, 00, 01, 03; W. 98, 99, 02, 03, 06)

☞ Teratogenicity: Teratogenicity is an ability of drug to induce foetal abnormality.

Teratogens: The substances which cause abnormalities of foetus development are called as teratogens, e.g. thalidomide, tetracyclines, diethylstilbesterol, penicillins, streptomycin, actinomycin-D.

Explanation

- Teratogens are the drugs or chemicals which if consumed by pregnant women then the effects are observed on foetus generally after birth.
- Teratogens affect somatic cells of foetus.
- Teratogens specifically affect the process of embryogenesis at a particular time of organogenesis, i.e. development of organs in foetus mainly from 7th week to 12th week of pregnancy in women.
- After fertilization of ovum till birth is called gestation period. This period is divided in 3 trimesters. The teratogen is administered during this period then adverse effects are observed on foetus and effects are dependant on duration and time of exposure to teratogens.
- Foetus is more susceptible than mother because cells of foetus mainly liver cells are not fully developed. If foetus is exposed to drug during first 10 to 12 weeks of gestation period, then toxicity is maximum.
- Teratogens in high doses in embryonic development can cause foetal death followed by abortion.
- **Factors affecting teratogenicity**
  - (i) Type of drug/teratogen
  - (ii) Time of exposure to the teratogen
  - (iii) Quantity of teratogen consumed by pregnant women.

Characteristics of Teratogenicity

1. **Specificity:** The teratogen effect if shown on one type of species then it may not be shown by other types of species, e.g. thalidomide is teratogenic on rabbits, man and not on rats.
2. **Time of exposure:** The teratogen effect is dependant on the time of exposure for teratogen during the gestation period. The teratogenic effect is shown by teratogen when exposure is in first trimester is not same when exposure is in last trimester, e.g. thalidomide.

Consumption period	**Effect**
(i) 21 to 22 days of gestation	• Absence of ears and paralysis of cranial nerve.
(ii) Upto 24 to 28 days of gestation	• Phocomelia may occur.

3. **Genotype of mother and foetus:** The teratogenic effect may be observed due to deficiency of any hormone, enzyme in mother and the sex of foetus also affects the toxicity of teratogen, e.g.
   (a) African people have deficiency of glucose-6-phosphate dehydrogenase and therefore, phenytoin toxicity may be observed.
   (b) If diethyl stilbesterol is consumed by pregnant women and foetus is female then at the teenage vaginal carcinoma may be observed.
4. **Simultaneous drug exposure:** When simultaneous exposure of drug and teratogen is observed, teratogenic effect may be observed, e.g. it folic acid antagonist is administered along with cortisone, facial abnormalities are observed in mice.
5. **Duration of exposure:** If large quantity of teratogen is consumed for longer period, teratogenic effect is observed in comparison with the consumption of teratogen by small quantity and for one or two times, e.g. thalidomide if consumed for only one time then phocomelia is not observed while if it is taken two times in between 4 to 7 weeks of pregnancy then phocomelia may occur.

List of Probable Teratogens and their Effects

Name of teratogen	Gestation period	Teratogenicity
1. Thalidomide (Hypnotic and sedative)	21 to 22 days	Absence of ears and paralysis of cranial nerves.
	24 to 27 days	Phocomelia (absence of arms and legs)
	28 to 29 days	Defects of legs.
2. Streptomycin		Deafness.
3. Stilbesterol		Vaginal carcinoma.

16

Drugs Used in Clinical Toxicity

1 Define and classify poisons with suitable examples. (S. 96, 97, 02, 05, 08, 09; W. 98, 00, 01, 03, 04, 08)

☞ Poison

"It is defined as a substance which when administered, inhaled, swallowed, applied locally, causes toxic effects on the body."

Classification of Poisons

A. **Irritant poisons**, e.g.
   (a) Organic, e.g. snake-venom
   (b) Inorganic, e.g. lead, mercury
   (c) Mechanical, e.g. glass powder

B. **Corrosive poisons**,e.g. conc. HCl, conc. H_2SO_4

C. **Neurotic poisons**, e.g. opium, strychnine

D. **Cardiac poisons**, e.g. digitalis

E. **Pulmonary poisons**, e.g. CO

F. **Miscellaneous** e.g. hallucinogens, antibiotics

(A) Irritant poisons: They produce symptoms of pain in the abdomen, vomiting, etc.

They are classified as:

(a) Organic irritants:
   (i) Vegetable, e.g. ergot
   (ii) Animal, e.g. snake-venom.

(b) Inorganic irritants:

(i) Metallic, e.g. lead, arsenic

(ii) Non-metallic, e.g. phosphorus.

(c) Mechanical irritants, e.g. glass powder.

(B) Corrosive poisons: A corrosive poison is simply a highly active irritant and not only produces inflammation but also acute ulceration of tissues.

They are classified as:

(i) Strong acids, e.g. H_2SO_4, HNO_3, HCl

(ii) Organic acids, e.g. oxalic acid, carbolic acid.

(iii) Concentrated alkalies, e.g. conc. NaOH, KOH

(C) Neurotic poisons: These poisons mainly act on CNS and may produce symptoms like headache, delirium, stupor, paralysis, coma, etc. For example, opium alkaloids, nuxvomica, conium and curare alkaloids.

(D) Cardiac poisons: These are acting on threat, e.g. digitals.

(E) Pulmonary poisons: These are affecting function of lung and interfere normal respiration, e.g. carbon monoxide.

(F) Miscellaneous poisons: These include hallucinogens, antibiotics, antihistaminics.

2 What are different types of poisonings?

☞ Types of Poisoning

(A) According to purpose of poisonings it is classified as:

(a) Suicidal poisoning: Person consumes poison to kill himself.

(b) Homicidal poisoning: Poison is used to kill another person.

(c) Accidental poisoning: The poison is consumed by mistake.

(B) On the basis of onset of action poisoning is classified into two groups:

(a) Acute poisoning

- It is generally due to consumption of a large amount of poison.
- It may be accidental, intentional or non-intentional.
- The symptoms develop very rapidly in severity.
- The aggravation of symptom is fast, therefore, treatment should be given quickly otherwise death may occur.
- The malfunctioning of respiratory and cardiac function causes further death.

- General symptoms of acute poisoning are vomiting, diarrhoea, convulsions, coma, respiratory or circulatory failure.
- It requires supportive, symptomatic and specific treatment.

(b) Chronic poisoning

- The symptoms are observed very slowly.
- It is due to consumption of small amount of poison but with definite period of interval.
- The aggravation of symptom is very slow.
- The death due to chronic poisoning is rarely observed because more time is available for the treatment.
- General symptoms of acute poisoning are GIT irritation, confusion, insomnia.
- Usually symptomatic treatment is given if required.

3 Define and classify antidotes with examples. (S. 06)

☞ Antidotes

The substances which stop the effects of poison are called antidotes.

Classification of Antidotes

1. **Physiological antidote:** It changes the physiology of body to prevent the effect of poison, e.g. sodium nitrite used in cyanide poisoning (dose 10 mg/kg).
2. **Chemical antidote:** It reacts with poison and converts it into non-poisonous compounds, e.g. sodium thiosulphate (dose 0.3–0.5 mg/kg).
3. **Mechanical antidote:** It prevents the absorption of poison, e.g. activated charcoal, kaolin.
4. **Universal antidote (*S. 04, 07; W. 05, 06*):** It is a combination of mechanical antidotes. It is useful when type of poison is not known or more than one poisons are consumed.

Composition of Universal Antidote

Magnesium oxide	1 Part (neutralizes acid)
Tannic acid	1 Part (precipitates alkaloids)
Activated charcoal	2 Parts (adsorbs alkaloid)

Dose

One to two tablespoonful should be taken with glass of water. The dose can be repeated after generally ½ hr interval till 4 to 6 hours.

Generally it is ineffective when poison is absorbed and the victim is unconscious.

4 Differentiate between acute poisoning and chronic poisoning. (S. 98, 99, 02, 04, 08; W. 99)

☞

Acute poisoning	Chronic poisoning
1. It is observed due to consumption of large amount of poisoning. 2. The symptoms observed are very fast. 3. The aggravation of symptoms is fast. 4. Death may occur. 5. Symptoms: vomiting, diarrhoea, convulsion, coma, respiratory or cardiac failure.	1. It is observed due to consumption of small amount of poison. 2. The symptoms observed are very slow. 3. The aggravation of symptoms is slow. 4. Death rarely occurs. 5. Symptoms: GIT irritation, confusion, coma, insomnia.

5 What are the steps involved in general treatment of poison? OR What are the principles of general treatment of poisoning? (S. 98, 01, 07, 08; W. 99, 08)

☞ The following are the steps involved in general treatment of poisoning:

1. Maintenance of normal respiratory and cardiac functions.
2. Removal of unabsorbed poison.
3. Removal of absorbed poison.
4. Use of antidotes.
5. Management of victim by treating general symptoms.

1. Maintenance of Normal Respiratory and Cardiac Functions

- For maintenance of normal respiratory and circulatory failure victim is first exposed to fresh air, if required artificial respiration is provided. Artificial respiration is adjusted by oxygen cylinders.
- To maintain the circulatory function CNS stimulants are used.
- CVS stimulants are also used if required.
- Respiratory stimulants like ammonium carbonate is given.

2. Removal of Unabsorbed Poison

- If poison is ingested orally, gastric lavage is performed to withdraw the gastric contents if the victim is conscious.

- By using emetics such as syrup of ipecac, mustard powder, etc. vomiting is induced to withdraw the contents in stomach.
- Mechanical antidotes like activated charcoal is used to adsorb poison on its surface mainly in case of alkaloidal poisoning.
- Gastric lavage is washing of stomach and it is useful only up to 4 to 6 hours after its consumption. In this method one tube is inserted into the stomach and by creating vacuum the contents are removed from GIT. This method is very useful in acid and alkaloidal poisoning because vomiting is not applicable for such poisoning treatment.
- To remove the poison from intestine purgatives like sodium or magnesium sulphate are used.
- If poison is inhaled then fresh air is used and artificial respiration is immediately given.
- If the poison is administered through skin, eye or wound then washing of skin or eye by plane warm water and also with water containing specific antidote is advisable.

3. Removal of Absorbed Poison

- The absorbed poison is prevented from its action by converting it into its non-poisonous form or by preventing binding of poison with specific receptors.
- Diuretics like manintol, frusemide are administered intravenously to increase excretion of poison.
- Hot packs are used to increase the sweating which helps to excrete the poisons through skin.
- Absorbed poison is removed by dialysis method. Dialysis may be peritoneal dialysis or haemodialysis.

4. Use of Antidotes

According to the type of poison and on the basis of route of administration of poison, antidote is selected.

Antidotes either react with poison or prevent binding of poison with receptor.

Common antidotes are sodium nitrite, EDTA, nalorphine, BAL.

5. Management of Victim by General Treatments

(i) In case of unconscious victim there is a maximum danger of respiratory infections, therefore, prophylactic antibiotics are used.

(ii) To avoid oedema diuretics are used.
(iii) To maintain glucose and ionic balance of blood, IV fluids are administered.
(iv) To treat weakness, food supplements, vitamins, iron are used.
(v) Hypotension is treated.
(vi) Analgesics are used as pain killers.
(vii) For restoring normal functioning of heart, cardiac stimulants are used.

6 Describe different poisoning along with their symptoms, treatments.

☞ 1. Mercury Poisoning

Symptoms	Treatments	Dose/Reason
a. **Acute poisoning**		
Metallic taste in mouth, grayish white tongue and mouth, nausea, vomiting,	• Egg albumin	Mechanical antidote
	• Charcoal pdr.	3 to 4 tablespoonful with water
cold skin, pale face, anorexia, dilated pupil,	• Stomach wash	With 5% solutions of sodium formaldehyde.
vomit with white mucus	• Dimercaprol	Systemic antidote
and blood, paralysis, renal failure, loss of weight, liver damage and shock.	• Peritoneal dialysis	To prevent renal failure
b. **Chronic poisoning**		
Multiple neurological disorders, irritability, shyness, loss of sleep, loss of memory, anxiety,	• Artificial respiration	Removal of patient from exposure and fresh air is provided to patient
tremors, hallucination, excessive salivation	• Penicillamine	Due to stable – SH gr. it is chelating agent.
with metallic taste, loosening of teeth with painful gums, colitis, hypertension, anaemia discolouration of lense	• Dimercaprol	Antidote. When dimercaprol is ineffective then penicillamine is a drug of choice.
of eye, renal failure, paralysis, coma,	• Dry extract of belladonna	30 mg 3 times a day promoting elimination of mercury by kidney and bowels.

Contd.

2. Cocaine Poisoning

Symptoms	Treatments	Dose/Reason
Mydriasis, dryness of mouth, increase in heart rate, hallucinations, black tongue, cyanosis, increase in nasal secretions.	• $KMnO_4$	Gastric lavage with $KMnO_4$ [1 : 100 diluted H_2O]
	• Artificial respiration	
	• Phenobarbitone	100 mg after every 4 hr orally
	• Tricyclic anti-depressants	As per requirements Washing of skin with water

3. Insecticide Poisoning (S. 99)

Insecticides are developed to kill insects and pests but they are absorbed from skin and GIT and are also toxic to human beings. They all are CNS stimulants and cause convulsions.

Symptoms	Treatments	Dose/Reason
Seizures similar to epilepsy with tremors, nausea, vomiting, ataxia, sensitization of myocardium leading to ventricular fibrillation, pulmonary oedema, liver and kidney damage, agranulocytosis	• Gastric lavage	To remove ingested poison. Skin is washed with soap and water if skin contamination is there.
	• Barbiturates (phenobarbitone 100 mg orally every 4 hr)	To control convulsions
	• Atropine	2 mg every 15 to 30 min by IM, IV.
	• Calcium acetate (10 ml of 10% solution)	Every 6 hr orally or IV to decrease toxicity of insecticides

4. Endrine Poisoning

Symptoms	Treatments	Dose/Reason
Nausea, vomiting, abdominal pains, salivation, convulsions,	• Barbiturates (phenobarbi-tone)	To control convulsions.

Contd.

Symptoms	Treatments	Dose/Reason
tremors, oozing of white froth form mouth and nostrils, coma, respiratory failure, death	• Calcium by IV	10 ml of 10% solution of calcium by IV after every 6 hr and calcium lactate orally decrease toxicity of endrine

5. Cannabis Poisoning

Symptoms	Treatments	Dose/Reason
Acute edema, excitement, depression, confusion, dilated pupil, drowsiness, hallucinations, increase in muscular movements, deep sleep, loss of weight, loss of appetite, weakness, tremors	• Stomach wash • Saline purgatives • Artificial respiration • Strychnine • Use of IV fluids	With water for removal of poison Hypodermal administration

6. Belladona Poisoning/Atropine Poisoning

Symptoms	Treatments	Dose/Reason
Dryness of mouth, bitter taste, abdominal pains, mydriasis, vomiting, delirium, fever, tachycardia, photophobia	• Stomach wash • Neostigmine/ physostigmine • Sponging • Diazepam	With 5% tannic acid As antidote To decrease body temperature 10 mg by IV

7. DDT Poisoning

Symptoms	Treatments	Dose/Reason
By contact: Tremors, convulsions, irritations of eye, nose, throat pulmonary edema, muscle spasms, paralysis of limb muscles, collapse and death.	• Barbiturates/ diazepam (phenobarbitone) • Gastric lavage • Saline cathartics	To control convulsions Stomach wash with water and antidote solution. To increase peristalsis movements and to

Contd.

Symptoms	Treatments	Dose/Reason
		excrete DDT without absorption.
By oral route: Salivation, nausea, vomiting, abdominal pain, tonic convulsions, tremors, hepatic cancer	• Antibiotic	To treat infection. Use of fat, oils should be avoided.

8. Opium Poisoning/Morphine/Narcotic Poisoning (S. 98, 05, 08)

Symptoms	Treatments	Dose/Reason
1. **Excitement:** Pleasurable mental excitement with increase in heart rate	• Stomach wash	With water and then with $KMnO_4$ at early stage
2. **Stupor:** Headache, itching, strong tendency to sleep, sense of weighing limbs, cyanosis of face and lips.	• Enema	Stomach wash is continued till returned water is of pink colour and then to clear intestine, enema is given
3. **Nacrosis:** Deep coma, relaxation of muscles, loss of reflexes, pin-point pupil, hypertension, low respiration, hypothermia, frothing from mouth	• Glucose saline, naloxone and nalorphine	5% Glucose with saline antidotes till dilation of pupils

9. Organophosphorous Poisoning

Symptoms	Treatments	Dose/Reason
1. Smooth muscles and glands are first affected and then brain centres are affected.	• Artificial respiration • Atropine	To block peripheral actions to counter, i.e. act muscarinic effects
2. Headache, constriction of chest with pin-point pupils	• Oxime compounds, e.g. pralidoxime	To control convulsions

Contd.

Symptoms	Treatments	Dose/Reason
3. Nausea, vomiting, diarrhoea, abdominal cramps, sweating, salivation, muscular switching.	• Antibiotics	To treat respiratory infections
4. Pulmonary edema, coma, convulsions, excessive bronchial secretions, bradycardia, respiratory failure.	• Mercurial diuretics	To avoid oedema.

10. Barbiturate Poisoning

Symptoms	Treatments	Dose/Reason
Nausea, mental confusion, depression, hypotension, skin rash, hypothermia, tremor, muscular weakness, in-coordination, stupor, edema, alternate contraction and relaxation of pupil, decreased urine output, drug automatism, respiratory failure, cold sweat breaks out	• Gastric lavage	With $KMnO_4$
	• Artificial respiration	
	• Metarminol IV	2.5 mg, to increase BP
	• Glucose saline	5% with saline for electrolyte balance and nutrition
	• Haemodialysis	For separation of poison
	• Forced diuresis	To increase urinary excretion
	• Enema	For removal of poison from GIT

11. Copper Poisoning

Symptoms	Treatments	Dose/Reason
Metallic taste, excessive salivation, abdominal pains, diarrhoea, green blue vomit, brown stools without blood, urine like ink and contains albumin.	• Stomach wash	With potassium salt
	• Charcoal powder	3 to 4 tablespoonful with water.
	• BAL	With usual dose as antidote.
Chronic symptoms: Hypertension, constipation, metallic taste, weakness, anorexia, headache		For chronic poisoning additionally belladona extract may be used.

Contd.

12. Arsenic Poisoning (W. 00, 05)

Symptoms	Treatments	Dose/Reason
(a) Acute: Capillary damage, epigastric and abdominal pains, vomiting, diarrhoea, jaundice, muscle cramps, pale face, dilated pupil, rapid pulse, convulsion, coma, death	• Artificial respiration	
	• Ferric oxide	To ppt. arsenic to harmless ferric arsenic
	• Sodium thiosulphate	By IV after every 46 hr
	• Dimercaprol (BAL)	Till the symptoms of arsenic disappear
	• Morphine	To reduce the pain.
(b) Chronic: Peripheral neuritis, diarrhoea, pigmentation of skin, liver damage, conjunctivitis oedema, carcinoma,	• Fresh air	Place the victim in fresh air
	• Sodium thiosulphate	By IV 1 gm in 10 ml water 2 to 3 times/ week for many weeks
1. Anorexia diarrhoea, occasional vomiting, fatigue	• Dimercoprol (BAL)	Till the control over arsenic symptoms
2. Conjunctivitis, eye and nose are affected, sense of fullness of head	• Anticonvulsants	To control convulsion
	• Antidiarrhoeals	To control diarrhoea.
3. Skin rash, brittle nails, failling of hairs		

13. Lead Poisoning (W. 99)

Symptoms	Treatments	Dose/Reason
(a) Acute: Metallic taste, vomiting, abdominal pains, constipation, suppressed urine, headache, black stools, loss of sleep, loss of vision, hallucination, delirium. convulsions,	• Stomach wash	10% $MgSO_4$ solution and then warm water. Repeated washing with regular interval
	• Penicillamine	Antidotes
	• Calcium EDTA	
(b) Chronic: Facial abnormalities, lead line on gums (blue line on gums) anaemia, constipation, paralysis of muscles, encephalopathy, hyperten-	• EDTA	Mixed with saline given by IV
	• BAL	For excretion of lead (in combination with EDTA it is more effective)

Contd.

Symptoms	Treatments	Dose/Reason
sion, menstrual disorders, abortion, nephritis, metallic taste, anorexia, weakness, headache		

7 Write a short note on "BAL"/"Dimercaprol". (S. 05, 06; W. 96)

- BAL means British Anti-Lewisite.
- It is also known as dimercaprol.
- Most of the enzymes in the body have –SH (mercapto) groups, which are essential for their activity. Many heavy metals like arsenic, mercury have a great affinity for these –SH groups.

Thus after combining with these –SH groups these compounds reactivate them.

- BAL has many –SH groups, which combine with these heavy metals leaving the –SH groups of enzymes of body free.
- The compound formed by heavy metal and di-thiol, dimercaprol is relatively stable and is excreted without causing damage to excretory mechanism (kidney, liver, etc.)

Preperations and Doses

(i) BAL is given intramuscularly as a 5% solution in arachis oil with benzyl benzoate.

(ii) BAL in the dose of 2.5–3 mg/kg administered by parenteral route.

BAL has considerable toxicities such as nausea, vomiting, burning sensation, anorexia, nephrotoxicity and hence should be used cautiously.

Uses of BAL/Dimercaprol

It is used as an antidote in metal poisoning due to antimony, arsenic, bismuth, gold, mercury, etc.

8 Mention the antidotes for different poisonings.

Poison	Antidote
1. Acid	CaO, MgO
2. Carbonic acid	$MgSO_4$
3. Lead	BAL, EDTA
4. Oxalic acid	Lime [$Ca(OH)_2$]
5. Phosphorus	Copper sulphate
6. Alkaloids	Tannins
7. Organophosphorus compounds	Atropine
8. Pilocarpine	Atropine
9. Morphine	Nalorphine, naloxone
10. Arsenic	BAL, EDTA
11. Copper	BAL, Penicillamine
12. Gold	BAL
13. Strychnine	Diazepam, chloroform,
14. Mercury	Penicillamine
15. Iron	Desferrioxime.
16. Barbiturate	Sodium bicarbonate.

17

Drug Abuse and Drug Dependence

1 Write a note on drug abuse. (S. 05, 07, 08; W. 04)

☞ Drug Abuse

The persistant and excessive use of drug apart from medical need is called drug abuse.

Drug Misuse

Improper use of drug is called drug misuse.

- Drug abuse causes harmful effects like habit, dependence and adverse effects.
- Drug misuse causes unwanted effects such as decrease in effectiveness or change in pharmacological effects.
- The drugs which are abused are as follows:

Classification of Drug Abuse

1. CNS depressants, e.g. alcohol, barbiturates, diazepam.
2. CNS stimulants, e.g. tobacco, amphetamine, cocaine.
3. Narcotics, e.g. morphine, heroin.
4. Volatile inhalants, e.g. acetone, benzene.
5. Hallucinogens, e.g. cannabis and its derivatives.

Reasons of Drug Abuse

1. The consumption for medicinal use.
2. To satisfy curiosity about drug effect.
3. To have new thrilling or dangerous experience.

4. To relax from stress and strain.
5. To escape from reality and to have a dreamy state.

Treatment of Drug Abuse (S. 08; W. 03)

Drug abuse treatment has two major dimensions:

1. Detoxification: It means freeing of the body from the adverse effects of the drug. It is done by stopping the drug and medical treatment for various withdrawal symptoms. It usually takes 10–21 days.
2. Rehabilitation: It is a long-term treatment. It involves psychotherapy, family therapy, behaviour therapy, group therapy.

2 What is drug dependence? Describe types of drug dependence. (S. 96, 01, 02, 03, 05; W. 96, 98, 02, 05)

☞ Drug Dependence

"It is a state of psychic also sometimes physical resulting from interaction between living organism and drug, showing behavioural and other responses and always include compulsion to take the drugs for getting experience of drugs psychic effect or to avoid discomfort."

Characteristics of any drug dependence are:

(i) Continuous desire of drug.
(ii) Periodic or regular intake.
(iii) Behavioral and other responses.
(iv) A tendency to increase the dose of a drug.
(v) Presence of withdrawal syndrome.

Examples of drugs forming dependence are alcohol, morphine, heroin, cannabis.

Types of Dependence

1. **Physical dependence:** It is defined as the condition in which the body "achieves" an adaptive state to the drug.
   - In this case the body shows intense physical disturbances when the drug is withdrawn.
   - The drug shows alteration at cellular level in CNS and causes development of tolerance which may further cause development of drug addiction.
   - Withdrawal symptoms may involve nausea, vomiting, diarrhoea, weakness, restlessness, dryness of mouth, etc.

- To treat withdrawal symptoms some another drugs may be used. Physical dependence is dependant on type of drug, quantity consumed and duration of use, e.g. to treat morphine addiction nalorphine is used.

Examples forming physical dependence: morphine, ethylalcohol, meprobamate.

2. **Psychic/Psychological dependence:** It is defined as a condition in which a drug produces a feeling of satisfaction and a psychic drive that requires periodic or continuous administration of the drug to produce pleasure or to avoid discomfort or anxiety. In this type of dependence there is no change in tissue or cells of the CNS, therefore, development of tolerance or resistant is not observed.
   - The withdrawal symptoms are less intense and usually non-toxic.
   - In this type of dependence there is no compulsion to take the drug therefore, this dependence is not difficult to treatment.

   Examples: caffeine, nicotine, cannabis, cocaine, LSD, mescaline.

Principles of Treatment of Drug Dependence

1. Gradual withdrawal of drug.
2. Substitution therapy.
3. Psychotherapy and occupational therapy.
4. Drug therapy.
5. Correction of dietary factors.
6. Community treatment.
7. Rehabilitation.
8. Expert guidance and specialized institutions are available for better treatment.

3 Differentiate between psychological dependence and physical dependence.

☞

Psychological dependence	Physical dependence
1. It is the condition in which a drug produces a feeling of satisfaction.	1. It is the condition in which the body achieves adaptive stage to the drug.
2. There is no compulsion to take the drug.	2. There is a compulsion to take the drug.

Contd.

Psychological dependence	Physical dependence
3. There is no withdrawal syndrome.	3. Intense withdrawal syndrome may occur.
4. Easy to treat psychic dependence.	4. Difficult to treat physical dependence.
5. Tolerance is not developed	5. Tolerance is developed.
6. Examples: caffeine, nicotine	6. Examples: morphine, alcohol.

4 Drug tolerance.

☞ **Definition:** "It is a state of decreased responsiveness to pharmacological effect of drug resulting from a prior exposure to that drug or related drugs."

Types of Tolerance

1. **Metabolic tolerance:** "It is due to increased deposition of drug on chronic use. The drug is further fastly metabolized, i.e. after chronic use, the cells of the body depend on drug."
2. **Behavioural tolerance:** "It is an ability to compensate the drug effect. It is dependant on physiology and ability of person."
3. **Functional tolerance:** "It is developed due to changes in receptor, enzymes or cell membranes for the action of drugs."
4. **Cross-tolerance:** "If one drug shows tolerance then other drugs belonging to same category also show tolerance."

5 Distinguish between drug habituation and drug addiction. (S. 96, 97, 99, 02, 08, 09; W. 98, 05)

☞

Drug habituation	Drug addiction
1. It is a condition resulting from repeated administration of the drug.	1. It is a state of periodic or chronic intoxication produced by repeated administration of drug.
2. It is accompanied with physiological dependence only.	2. It is accompanied with physical and psychological dependence.
3. Tolerance is not developed.	3. Tolerance is developed.

Contd.

Drug habituation	Drug addiction
4. No tendency to increase dose of a drug.	4. Tendency to increase the dose for getting satisfaction of drug effects.
5. Withdrawal symptoms are not severe and are very less.	5. Withdrawal symptoms are severe and require medical treatment. Sometimes hospitalisation is needed.
6. Person has strong desire to get drug.	6. Person shows compulsion to take drug.
7. No detrimental effects on society.	7. Detrimental effects on both person and society.
8. Examples: tea, coffee.	8. Examples: morphine, alcohol.

6 What is addiction? Name three drugs which cause addiction. How is it treated? (S. 01, 07; W. 02)

☞ Addiction

"A continuous administration of certain drugs forces the person to use more doses and tendency to increase the dose and high tendency to withdrawal effects is known as drug addition."

Drugs causing addiction are morphine, heroin, cannabis, alcohol.

Causes/Reasons of Drug Addiction

1. The consumption for medicinal use.
2. To satisfy curiosity about drug effect.
3. To have new thrilling or dangerous experience.
4. To relax from stress and strain.
5. To escape from reality.
6. To have a dreamy state.

Treatments of Drug Addiction

1. Gradual withdrawal of drug.
2. Substitution therapy.
3. Psychotherapy and occupational therapy.
4. Drug therapy.
5. Correction of dietary/nutritional factors.
6. Community treatment.

7. Rehabilitation.
8. Expert guidance and specialized institutions are available for better treatment.

7 Write a note on "hallucinogens". (S. 02. 08)

☞ **Hallucinogens**

Hallucinogens are the drugs that act on CNS to produce a state of perception of objects with no reality. They are also called psychotomimetics, e.g. LSD (lysergic acid diethylamide), mescaline.

LSD is the most common hallucinogen of abuse. 20 to 25 μg of LSD may produce effects in susceptible individuals and may last for 8–12 hr.

Major Effects of LSD

Blurred vision, altered shapes and colours, sounds may be seen, distortion of space, hallucination, dizziness, muscular weakness, increased HR, dry mouth, nausea, vomiting, tremors. Psychological changes show altered moods, euphoria, decreased ability to concentrate, tension, anxiety.

Treatments for patients taking LSD

1. Supportive environment.
2. Use of antianxiety and sedative drugs.
3. Use of antipsychotics for schizophrenic patients.

8 Write a note on alcohol addiction/alcoholism. OR Write a note on medical complications, withdrawal symptoms and treatments of alcoholism.

☞
- Alcoholism is a behavioural disorder and a chronic disease state resulting due to persistent and excessive use of alcohol.
- It causes physical disability and impaired emotional, occupational and interpersonal adjustment.
- Alcohol addiction involves both tolerance and physical dependence.
- Medical complication of alcoholism: It includes, malabsorption, gastritis, cirrhosis, alcoholic hepatitis, fatty liver, chronic diarrhoea, beriberi, cutaneous ulcers, delirium, tremors, convulsions, pellagra, hypo- or hyperglycemia.
- Withdrawal symptoms of alcoholism: Sweating, insomnia, headache, muscle twitching, tachycardia, diarrhoea, vomiting, agitation, hallucinations, disorientation.

Treatments of Alcoholism

1. To overcome nutritional deficiencies give vitamin B mainly thiamine (B_1) and nicotinic acid (B_3).
2. Intravenous fluid and electrolyte replacement is also recommended.
3. Sedatives like chlordiazepoxide, diazepam may be given.
4. Supportive psychotherapy.
5. Drugs like disulfiram (antidote) in dose 0.5 gm/day is used.
6. Metronidazole is used to control diarrhoea.
7. Long-term management: Participation in supportive social organizations to overcome alcoholism.
8. Psychiatric therapy.

9 Elaborate important drug of abuses, withdrawal symptoms and treatments.

☞ **1. Barbiturate Addiction**

Symptoms	Drug used	Dose/Reason
Anxiety, confusion, delirium, anorexia, insomnia, muscular pains, nausea, abdominal cramps, disorientation and coma.	(a) Phenobarbitone (b) Antihistaminics or phenothiazines	For stabilization of patient. To avoid development of drug seeking behaviour. Psychotherapy. Gradual withdrawal of drug over a period of ten days to minimize withdrawal symptoms.

2. Amphetamine Addiction

Symptoms	Drug used	Dose/Reason
Depression, fatigue muscular pains, hypersomnia, renal failure, Intracranial haemorrhage, hypertension.	(a) Tranquillizers (b) Haloperidol (c) Tricyclic antidepressants (d) IV fluid	To reduce craving To treat symptomatic stimulation. To treat prolonged depression. For replacement therapy.

3. Cocaine Addiction

Symptoms	Drug used	Dose/Reason
Anxiety, irritability, visual disturbances, weight loss, nausea, hallucinations,	(a) Tranquillizers (b) CVS drugs	To reduce craving. To regulate function of CVS and rest.

Contd.

Symptoms	Drug used	Dose/Reason
insomnia, cardiac arrhythmia, muscular pains, depression.	(c) Tricyclic antidepressants.	To treat prolonged depression. Psychological treatment.

4. Hallucinogen/Psychotomimetic Addiction

Symptoms	Drug used	Dose/Reason
Dryness of mouth, confusion, disorientation, muscular pains, tremors inco-ordination, acute leukaemia, tachycardia, abnormality in eye, nausea, vomiting, altered moods, euphoria, tension, anxiety.	(a) Chlorpromazine (b) Diazepam	To reduce craving. To treat tremor and extreme agitation. Psychotherapy. Rehabilitation. Symptomatic and replacement treatment is required.

5. Tobacco Addiction

Symptoms	Drug used	Dose/Reason
Disorientation, dryness of mouth, tachycardia, tremors, leukaemia, lung cancer, hypertension, irritability, anxiety, insomnia, headache.	(a) Clonidine (b) Haloperidol (c) IV fluids	To treat hypertension. To treat sympathomimetic stimulation For replacement therapy. Symptomatic and supportive treatment. Psychotherapy.

6. Narcotic Addiction/Opioid Addiction (S. 99, 01, 05; W. 02)

Symptoms	Drug used	Dose/Reason
Sudden withdrawal causes:		
(a) After 8 hr: Anxiety, yawning, sneezing, tearing	(a) Methadone (as substitute)	20 mg in divided doses for 1st three days and then 10 mg for next 3 days.
(b) After 20 hr: Sweating, pains.	(b) LAAM (levo alpha acetyl methadone)	LAAM is superior than methadone and administered daily.
(c) After 24–48 hr: Nausea, vomiting, diarrhoea, fever hypertension.	(c) Clonidine (d) Opioid antagonists such as naloxone,	To treat hypertension. To counter narcotic effects.

Contd.

Symptoms	Drug used	Dose/Reason
(d) Up to 1 week: Muscle cramps.	nalorphine	
(e) Up to several months insomnia, bradycardia, pulmonary oedema cardiorespiratory collapse, hepatitis, tremors, muscle spasms, GIT cramps, bodyaches, malnutrition leading to dehydration, acid-base disturbances. Infection of AIDS may cause.	(e) Antibiotics (f) Analgesics	To treat respiratory infections. To treat pains. Psychotherapy Rehabilitation Correction of malnutrition deficiencies.

7. Alcohol Addiction (S. 06, 09; W. 08)

Symptoms	Drugs used	Treatments
(a) Acute alcohol addiction:	(a) Artificial respiration	To maintain respiratory function
20 mg: Feeling of wrath 30 mg: Relief from anxiety	(b) Electrolytes	To maintain body temperature.
50 mg: In-coordination, slurring of speech.	(c) Hypertonic mannitol solution	To decrease intracranial pressure
100–200 mg: Vomiting, imbalance, ataxia, muscular in-coordination.	(d) Phenothiazine	To control psychic behaviour
300 mg: Stuper 400 mg: Respiratory depression.	(e) Disulfiram	Antidote of alcoholism.
(b) Chronic alcohol addiction:	(a) Diazepam 40 mg daily for 4 days	To treat craving.
Tremors, anxiety,	(b) Metronidazole	Antidiarrhoeal
insomnia, confusion	(c) Haloperidol	To treat convulsions
gastritis, hepatitis, peptic ulcer, sweating, fever, pancreatitis, convulsions, bone marrow depression, tachycardia, diarrhoea.	(d) Vitamin B complex	To overcome nutritional deficiencies mainly thiamine and nicotinic acid. Psychotherapy Rehabilitation For long-term management participation in supportive social organizations to overcome alcoholism.

18

Bioavailability of Drugs

1 Define bioavailability. Give types of bioavailability. (S. 96, 97, 99, 00, 01, 02, 03; W. 96, 98, 01)

☞ Bioavailability

"It is defined as the rate and extent at which active concentration of drug is available at the desired site of action."

Types of Bioavailability

1. **Relative bioavailability:** The relative bioavailability is the bioavailability in comparison with reference standard.
2. **Absolute bioavailability:** The absolute bioavailability is the bioavailability in which whole quantity of administered drug reaches the blood circulation." It is possible only by IV route.

2 Define 'bioequivalence'. Give its types. (S. 05, 09; W. 96, 99, 04)

☞ Bioequivalence

If two or more similar dosage forms of same drug reach in blood circulation at the same relative rate and to same relative extent under the same experimental conditions, then those preparations are called bioequivalent preparations.

Types of Bioequivalence

1. **Clinical equivalence:** "The two brand products of one drug are said to be clinically equivalent if they produce same

pharmacological response under the same experimental conditions and same objects."

2. **Chemical equivalence:** "If two or more dosage forms of the same drug contain same labelled quantities of drug, then those preparations are called a chemical equivalent preparations."
3. **Therapeutic equivalence:** "If structurally different drugs provide the same therapeutic or clinical response under same experimental conditions then those drugs are said to be therapeutically equivalent."

3 Give the importance or object of studying bioavailability.

☞ **Study of bioavailability is necessary:**

1. To avoid toxic and side effects of the drugs.
2. To adjust the dosage regimen.
3. To study pharmacological action of drug.
4. For pre-formulation study.
5. To judge about the clinical responses of drugs.
6. To avoid wastage of dugs.
7. To decide the dose and dosage forms.

4 Enumerate different factors that affect/influence the bioavailability of a drug. (S. 96, 97, 98, 99, 00, 01, 02; W. 96, 98, 99, 01, 02, 04, 08)

☞

Factors affecting bioavailability of drug		
(a) Pharmaceutical factors	**(b) Physiological factors**	**(c) Physicochemical factors**
Dosage form Dissolution rate Manufacturing variables	Anatomy of GIT Gastric emptying rate Gastric pH Food Interaction with GI components First pass effect Diseased condition Drug-durg interaction GIT flora	Particle size Stability Complex formation Viscosity Surfactants P^{KA} and P^{KB} Partition coefficient Salt form Particle state Molecular weight Route of administration of drug.

5 Explain different pharmaceutical factors affecting bioavailability of drug. (S. 00, 07; W. 96, 98, 99, 02, 06)

1. Dosage Form

- Various types of dosage forms of drugs are available.
- The bioavailability of drug is dependant on rate of dissolution, absorption, distribution, elimination process.
- The bioavailability of dosage forms is as follows: Injection > Solution > Suspension > Powder > Capsule > Tab > Coated tablets.

2. Dissolution Rate

If the dissolution rate is more then rate of absorption is increased thus bioavailability is more.

Dissolution rate is calculated by Noyes-Whiney equation:

$$\text{Dissolution rate} = \frac{DAK\,[C_s - C_b]}{h}$$

Where, D = Diffusion coefficient
C_s = Conc. of drug in stagnant layer
C_b = Conc. of drug in solvent
A = Surface area
K = Partition coefficient
h = Thickness of stagnant layer.

Thus, dissolution rate is directly proportional to surface area, partition coefficient and inversely proportional to thickness of stagnant layer (h).

3. Manufacturing Variables

Various additives are used during the preparation of dosage forms. Different processes such as mixing, granulation, drying, compression, are followed during preparation of dosage forms.

Thus additives and process of manufacturing may affect the bioavailability of a drug, e.g.

(i) Lubricants are hydrophobic, therefore, bioavailability of drug gets decreased if lubricant used is more.

(ii) If the force of compression is increased during the tablet preparation then the hardness of tablet is more therefore, disintegration of tablet is more and thus bioavailability is decreased.

(iii) If the amount of binder is more during preparation of tablet, then it is very difficult to disintegrate or dissolve. Thus rate of absorption is decreased and bioavailability is decreased.

6 Explain different physiological factors affecting bioavailability of drug. (S. 03, 05, 08, 09; W. 01)

☞1. **Anatmoy of GIT:** Absorbing surface area of stomach is lesser as compared to small intestine. The absorption of the drug is more in its unionized form, therefore, acidic drugs are well absorbed in stomach and basic drugs well absorbed through intestine.
   For example, the salicylates, barbiturates are well absorbed through stomach than through intestine.
   Ephedrine, pethidine are well absorbed through intestine than through stomach.
2. **Gastric emptying rate:** It is the time required for emptying 50% material to pass through GIT. It is affected by temperature and anatomy of the person and volume of material.
   Anticholinergic drugs are parasympatholytic therefore, PSNS gets depressed therefore, gastric emptying rate is decreased and due to depression of function of absorbing cells of the GIT, the bioavailability gets decreased.
3. **Gastric pH:** Acidic drugs are in unionized from in stomach therefore, these are well absorbed in stomach due to acidic nature of stomach content and similarly basic drugs are well absorbed in intestine.
4. **Food:** Presence of food in GIT reduces absorption of amoxicillin, ampicillin. While in presence of food side effects of some drugs like iron, such as GIT irritation, vomiting, nausea, are reduced. The iron compounds are if taken on empty stomach then nausea, vomiting may be observed and if taken along with food then their absorption is reduced. Therefore, the drugs are taken half an hour after the meal.
5. **Interaction with GI components**
   - Bile salts reaction with antibacterial agents and inactivate them and therefore, their absorption is less.
   - Bile salts enhance dissolution of poorly soluble drugs and thus bioavailability is more.
   - The innermost wall of GIT forms a binding with streptomycin and gentian violet and thus their bioavailability is reduced.
   - Insulin is inactivated by acidity in stomach therefore, its bioavailability by oral route is nearly zero.

7 Explain physicochemical properties/factors affecting bioavailability of drug. (S. 99; W. 96, 02, 03)

☞1. **Particle size:** Smaller the particle size of drug, greater is the absorption of drug. Thus bioavailability is increased. Thus capsules have more bioavailability than tablets.
2. **Stability:** Insulin and penicillin are unstable in acidic medium because these drugs are inactivated by acidity of stomach. Penicillin-G is also unstable in aqueous medium. Therefore, its injection should be freshly prepared before its administration.
3. **Complex formation:** Streptomycin and gention violet form a binding with innermost wall of GIT. They react with mucin to form a complex and thus bioavailability is reduced.
   Tetracyclines when administered with milk form a complex with calcium in the milk. Thus reduce absorption of tetracycline and reduce bioavailability.
4. **Viscosity:** Gastric emptying rate of viscous liquids is more, therefore, greater is the absorption and bioavailability is more. The viscous liquids remain at site of absorption for more time. Therefore, generally cough syrups are preferred as expectorants. Non-viscous liquids have less bioavailability.
5. **Surfactants:** Surfactants reduce the interfacial tension and therefore, absorption of drug is increased and bioavailability is increased.
6. **First-pass effect:** "It is the time required for the drug to pass through hepatic portal system." Thus rate of metabolism is related with this time. After metabolism drug is inactivated therefore, the bioavailability of such drug is reduced.
7. **Diseased condition:** In dysentery and diarrhoea, motility of GIT is increased therefore, in such disorder, if drug is given by oral route then absorption of drug is less therefore, bioavailability of drug is reduced. If the person is suffering form kidney or liver disorders then rates of elimination and metabolism are changed and therefore, bioavailability is affected.
8. **Drug-drug interaction:** Simultaneous administration of two drugs may change the absorption of any one or both drugs, e.g. liquid paraffin decreases absorption of vitamin A.
9. **GIT flora:** Disturbances in normal flora of GIT lead to disturbances in absorption of drug and thus affect bioavailability.

Board Question Papers

(From Summer 1996 to Summer 2017)

Summer Examination 1996

D Pharm Second Year

Hospital and Clinical Pharmacy

Q 1. Solve any *five* of the following:

a. Explain the following terms (any *four*):
   i. Etiology
   ii. Pathogenosis
   iii. Lesion
   iv. Fortis
   v. Tussis

b. Translate into English (any *four*):
   i. BIS
   ii. Libra
   iii. Parvus
   iv. Secundus
   v. Folium

c. What advice must be given to the patients using (any *four*):
   i. Salicylate
   ii. Ampicillin
   iii. Phenolphthalein
   iv. Boric acid
   v. Sulfa drugs

d. Differentiate between drug addiction and drug habituation.

e. Fill in the blanks:
   i. DIS and DIC stands for ________ and ________ respectively.
   ii. ________ is the drug used to treat TB but induces ________.
   iii. Number of rabbits used for pyrogen test when it is repeated second time is ________.
   iv. In case of ________ type of epilepsy unconsciousness last for longer time.
   v. Normal haemoglobin content per gram in female is ________.

f. Give normal values and significance of (any *two*):
   i. RBC count
   ii. Blood sugar
   iii. Eosinophils

g. Define the following terms (any *four*):
   i. Drug-dependance
   ii. Hypotensives
   iii. Immunity
   iv. Sterilisation
   v. Elixirs

Q 2. Answer any *four* of the following:

a. Define out-patient, emergency out-patient and in-patient.
b. Give short account of hospitals classified on the basis of ownership.
c. Give benefits of unit dose system.
d. Define hospital and classify it with suitable examples.
e. What is bed-side pharmacy? Give its importance.
f. Give objectives of hospital pharmacy.

Q 3. Answer any *four* of the following:

a. How dispensing of charged non-floor stock is carried out?
b. What are the sources of collection of information?
c. Name three surgical instruments with their uses.
d. What economic consideration governs the decision of make or buy drug in hospital pharmacy?
e. Draw floor plan of sterile product area.
f. Give conditions to be fulfilled by all parenteral preparations.

Q 4. Solve any *four* of the following:

a. Give functions of pharmacy and therapeutic committee.
b. Describe safety test to be performed in transfusion and infusion assemblies as per IP 1985.
c. Name various standards prescribed by IP for purity of absorbent cotton.
d. Give use of following:
   i. Glucometer
   ii. Laminar-flow
   iii. ECG machine
e. Define hospital formulary and give guideline while using it.
f. Define clinical pharmacy and describe its scope.

Q 5. Solve any *four* of the following:

a. Give normal values of:
   i. Cholesterol
   ii. WBC count
   iii. ESR
   iv. Specific gravity of urine
   v. Pulse rate
   vi. Respiration rate
b. Write a note on surgical dressings.
c. Define bioavailability and name various factors affecting it.
d. Give causes of adverse drug reactions.

e. What is food drug interaction? Explain with example.
f. Classify poisons with examples.

Q 6. Solve any *four* of the following:

a. Give composition of universal antidote and mention its uses.
b. Define drug interaction and name types of drug interaction mechanisms.
c. Write a note on idiosyncrasy or teratogenicity.
d. Describe signs and symptoms of tuberculosis (TB)
e. Write a note on health delivery system in India.
f. Give application of computer in maintenance of records in hospitals.

Winter Examination 1996

D Pharm Second Year

Hospital and Clinical Pharmacy

Q 1. Solve any *five* of the following:

a. Give normal values and significance of (any *two*):
   i. Cholesterol
   ii. Heart rate
   iii. Basophils
b. Define the following (any *four*):
   i. Sterilisation
   ii. Eyedrops
   iii. Ointments
   iv. Elixirs
   v. Creams
c. Explain the following (any *four*):
   i. Prescription
   ii. Amoebiasis
   iii. Anaesthetics
   iv. Counter irritants
   v. Laxatives
d. Name the method or methods of sterilisation used to sterilise (any *four*):
   i. Rubber gloves
   ii. Metal needles
   iii. Absorbent cotton
   iv. Plastic wound dressings
   v. Glassware
e. Differentiate between:
   i. Sympathetics and parasympathetics.
   ii. Sympatholytics and parasympatholytics.
f. What advice must be given to the patient using (any *four*):
   i. Liquid paraffin
   ii. Boric acid
   iii. Tetracycline
   iv. Antidiabetics
   v. Purgatives

g. Translate into English (any *four*):

i. Tussis
ii. Secundus
iii. Gutta
iv. Libra
v. Die

Q 2. Answer any *four* of the following:

a. Write short account of the hospitals classified on the basis of size.
b. What are requirements and abilities of hospital pharmacist?
c. How will you decide the location of hospital pharmacy.
d. Write short note on prepackaging.
e. What do you mean by bedside pharmacy?
f. Give criteria for selecting the noncharge floor stock drug.

Q 3. Answer any *four* of the following:

a. What is the role of pharmacist in improving patient compliance?
b. What is central service? Which departments are served by the central service?
c. Explain how flow of materials takes place in sterile area.
d. Name the types of additives added to parenteral products.
e. Write about tender system purchasing in hospitals.
f. Name three types of scissors and their uses.

Q 4. Solve any *four* of the following:

a. How entry and deletion of drugs in the hospital formulary is done?
b. What is the purpose of establishing drug information services?
c. Write short note on information retrival by computers.
d. How PTC is constituted?
e. What is purchase requisition?
f. What is nonsterile manufacture? How suppositories are prepared by fusion process?

Q 5. Answer any *four* of the following:

a. Define and classify adverse drug reaction.
b. What is drug-food interaction? Explain with example.
c. Give the meaning and importance of clinical pharmacy.
d. Mention the use of dimercaprol and EDTA in the treatment of poisoning.
e. Define drug dependance and give its types.
f. Give reasons for drug abuse.

Q 6. Answer any *four* of the following:

a. Define:

i. Bioavailability
ii. Bioequivalence
iii. Absolute bioavailability

b. Discuss various pharmaceutical factors affecting bioavailability of the drug.
c. Give different subdivisions of sterile area.
d. What are surgical dressings? How are they sterilised?
e. Give objectives of hospital pharmacy.
f. What is the purpose of medical records? Give its principles.

Summer Examination 1997

D Pharm Second Year

Hospital and Clinical Pharmacy

Q 1. Solve any *five* of the following:

a. What advice must be given to the patients using (any *four*):
   i. Diazepam
   ii. Salicylate
   iii. Chloramphenicol
   iv. Phenolphthalein
   v. Sulfa drugs

b. Translate into English (any *four*):
   i. Cataplasma
   ii. Succus
   iii. Semel
   iv. Ter
   v. Unus

c. Explain the following terms (any *four*):
   i. Emetics
   ii. Analeptics
   iii. Immunity
   iv. Cholagogue
   v. Tranquilizers

d. Define the following terms (any *four*):
   i. Tablets
   ii. Tinctures
   iii. Elixirs
   iv. Emulsions
   v. Capsules

e. Write at least four points of difference between drug addiction and drug habituation.

f. Fill in the blanks:
   i. The ________ committee suggested that hospital should have manufacturing facilities for IV fluids.
   ii. The most extensively used antioxidant is ________.
   iii. ________ decreases toxicity of endrin.
   iv. Five healthy ________ are used for carrying out safety test, weighing approximately ________ g.

g. Give normal values and significance of (any *two*):
   i. Haemoglobin
   ii. ESR
   iii. RBC

Q 2. Answer any *four* of the following:

a. Define and classify hospitals.
b. Name different drug distribution systems in hospitals and define emergency out-patients and in-patients.
c. Give benefits of unit dose system.
d. Give various administrative patterns of central services.
e. Write a short note on laminar air flow.
f. What is manufacture of drugs? Name the equipments for manufacture of tablets.

Q 3. Answer any *four* of the following:

a. Give methods of estimating demand of hospitals.
b. What is clinical pharmacy? State its importance in short.
c. Name any three:
   i. Preservatives used in injectables.
   ii. Tonicity contributors for injectables.
d. Define hospital formulary and give its significance.
e. What are the qualifications of pharmacist to run drug information service?
f. Explain the use of computers in inventory control, in a drug-store.

Q 4. Answer any *four* of the following:

a. What is tuberculosis (TB) and mention drugs used to control/treat them?
b. Give functions of PTC.
c. Name types of glass used to prepare container. Explain principle involved in hydrolytic resistance test for glass containers.
d. Write short note on drug-information bulletin.
e. What is general procedure for production of syrup?
f. What is purchase requisition? To whom it is sent for procurement?

Q 5. Answer any *four* of the following:

a. Define drug interaction. Give types and mechanism of drug interaction.
b. Define and classify adverse drug reaction.
c. What are surgical dressings? Give its uses.
d. Give treatments of drug abuse.
e. Define bioavailability and name factors affecting it.
f. What are surgical instruments? Name any three with uses.

Q 6. Answer any *four* of the following:

a. Give functions of hospital pharmacy.
b. What is a bed-side pharmacy?

c. Give classification of poisons with suitable examples.
d. What are the economic consideration which governs the decisions of make or buy in hospital pharmacy?
e. What are various additives in the parenterals?
f. Differentiate between psychologic and physical drug dependance.

Summer Examination 1998

D Pharm Second Year

Hospital and Clinical Pharmacy

Q 1.

a. **Attempt any *three* of the following:**
   i. Define hospital
   ii. What is bed-side pharmacy?
   iii. What is laminar flow?
   iv. Define hospital pharmacy.

b. What are the qualities required by a pharmacist to run the drug information service?

Or

What are surgical instruments? Name any five surgical instruments and the purpose for which they are used.

Q 2. Answer any *four* of the following:

a. What are surgical dressings? How are they qualified? Describe the test for identity for absorbent cotton.
b. State how computers are useful in the purchase and inventory control of medicaments.
c. Explain the significance of hospital formulary system.
d. Describe why and how pharmacy and therapeutics committee is formulated.
e. What do you mean by centralised or decentralised purchases? Describe to whom the copies of purchase orders are given and why?

Q 3. Attempt any *four* of the following:

a. What is nonsterile manufacture of drugs? Desceibe the requirements of tablet-section.
b. What are the functions of modern hospitals?
c. What are the requirements of space and equipments for the smooth and normal working of a hospital?
d. Describe the administrative and technical qualities required by a pharmacist.

e. Who is an administrator of a hospital? What functions he has to perform?

Q 4.

a. **Answer any *three* of the following:**
   i. What do you mean by clinical pharmacy?
   ii. What is patient counselling?
   iii. What do you mean by analgesics and antipyretics?
   iv. What are generic names?
   v. Define drug interactions.

b. Name and discuss three physiological factors which affect the bioavailability of drugs.

Or

Differentiate between the psychologic drug dependance and physical drug dependance with suitable examples.

Q 5. Answer any *four* of the following:

a. Differentiate acute and chronic poisoning.
b. What are adverse drug reactions? How are they classified?
c. What are drug interactions? Write a note on pharmacodynamic interactions of drugs.
d. What are physiological parameters? Do they help in diagnosis of diseases. Explain with two suitable examples.
e. Write a note on signs and symptoms of tuberculosis.

Q 6.

a. Describe in short the steps involved in the treatment of poisons.
b. Write short notes on any two:
   i. Hallucinogens
   ii. Pathophysiology of diabetes
   iii. Importance of DLC

Winter Examination 1998

D Pharm Second Year

Hospital and Clinical Pharmacy

Q 1.

a. **Attempt any *three* of the following:**
   i. Name various systems of classifying the hospitals.
   ii. Classify various types of out-patients.
   iii. Define unit-dose dispensing.
   iv. What is bed-side pharmacy?

b. Discuss the factors affecting make or buy decision to undertake the manufacturing in hospitals.

Or

Describe in short, how drugs are distributed to in-patients in a typical hospital?

Q 2. Answer any *four* of the following:

a. Name various sub-divisions of manufacture in sterile area and describe their purpose in short.

b. What is manufacture of drugs? Describe various requirements to undertake the manufacture of tablets or suppositories in an hospital.

c. What is pharmacy and therapeutics committee? Name its important functions.

d. What is hospital formulary system? State the importance of having hospital formulary.

e. What are surgical dressings? Name the various pharmacopoeial tests to be performed on absorbent cotton wool IP.

Q 3. Attempt any *four* of the following:

a. What is information retrieval by computers? State the importance of drug information retrieval.

b. What is drug information service? What are the sources of collecting the drug informations?

c. Write a short note on drug information bulletin.

d. What are surgical instruments? Name any three instruments used for surgical operations and their respective uses.

e. Write a note on abilities of a pharmacist.

Or

Describe the obejctives of hospital pharmacy services.

Q 4.

a. **Answer any *three* of the following:**

i. What is clinical pharmacy?

ii. How will you advise the patient regarding the proper storage of drugs?

iii. Define haematinics with suitable examples.

iv. What are OTC products?

v. Define bioavailability of drugs.

b. Discuss various factors affecting the bioavailability of drugs.

Or

Distinguish between drug addiction and drug habituation with suitable examples.

Q 5. Answer any *four* of the following:

a. What are adverse drug reactions? Discuss three adverse drug reactions.

b. Name the various types of dosage forms which are labelled as "for external use only" or "shake well before use". Explain the importance of these instructions.

c. Describe the signs and symptoms of tuberculosis or hepatitis.

d. What is significance of RBC or WBC count?

e. Write a note on drug-food infection.

Q 6.

a. What are poisons? How are they classified? Quote suitable examples. Describe the steps involved in the treatment of poisoning.

b. Write short notes on any two:

i. Hypertension

ii. Teratogenicity

iii. Drug-dependance

Summer Examination 1999

D Pharm Second Year

Hospital and Clinical Pharmacy

Q 1. Attempt the following:

a. Define (any *two*):

i. Adverse drug-reaction

ii. Manufacture of drugs

iii. Bioavailability of drugs

b. What do you mean by (any *four*):

i. Haematinics

ii. Anaesthetics

iii. Analeptics

iv. Immunity

v. Astringents

vi. Sialogogue

c. Define the following (any *four*):

i. Suppositories

ii. Capsules

iii. Poultices

iv. Elixirs

v. Tinctures

vi. Liquid orals

d. Mention the suitable method of sterilisation of the following with reason to prefer the method (any *two*):

i. Intramuscular oily injection

ii. Surgical dressings

iii. Plastic containers used for saline solution.

e. Give the noraml values of (any *four*):
   i. Blood sugar
   ii. Cholesterol
   iii. Pulse rate in adult males
   iv. RBC
   v. Basophils

Q 2. Attempt any *two* of the following:

a. Discuss the physical properties of the drug which affect their bio-availability.
b. Describe the functions of a hospital pharmacy.
c. Describe the various methods of procurement of medicaments in hospital store.

Q 3. Write short notes on (any *three*):

a. Bed-side pharmacy
b. Drug-food interaction
c. Treatment of insect-poisoning
d. Drug-abuse
e. Out-patient services.

Q 4. What do you know about (any *three*):

a. Functions of pharmacy and therapeutic committee.
b. Testing of pharmaceutical raw materials in hospital pharmacy.
c. Machinery and equipment required for manufacture of tablets.
d. Unit dose system.

Q 5.

a. Describe the symptoms and pathophysiology of diabetes of peptic ulcer.
b. Explain how computers help in drug-information retrieval and storage.

Or

Write short note on medication monitoring and drug-information.

Q 6. Attempt any *four* of the following:

a. Differentiate between drug habituation and drug addiction.
b. What is chronic poisoning? How arsenic poisoning is treated?
c. What is drug-induced gastrointestinal toxicity, explain with suitable examples.
d. What advice a pharmacist should offer to the patient in the treatment with the following drugs (any *two*):
   i. Haematinics
   ii. Vaginal contraceptive suppositories
   iii. Chloramphenicol

e. What are objectives of clinical pharmacy?
f. Explain the narcotic drugs with their advantage and disadvantage.

Winter Examination 1999
D Pharm Second Year
Hospital and Clinical Pharmacy

Q 1. Attempt any *five* of the following:

a. Define (any *two*):
   i. Bioequivalence
   ii. Bioavailability of drug
   iii. Hospital formulary system
b. What do you mean by (any *four*):
   i. Tranquilizers
   ii. Purgatives
   iii. Cathartics
   iv. Carminatives
   v. Demulscents
   vi. Emetics
c. Define the following (any *four*):
   i. Lotions
   ii. Capsulcs
   iii. Vehicles
   iv. Pastes
   v. Emulsions
   vi. Ointments
d. Mention the suitable method of sterilization of the following with reason to prefer the method (any *two*):
   i. Hand gloves
   ii. Surgical instruments
   iii. Normal saline for injection
e. Give the noraml values of (any *four*):
   i. Clotting time of blood
   ii. RBC
   iii. Respiration rate per minute in adult male

Q 2. Answer any *two* of the following:

a. Discuss the pharmaceutical factors which affect the bioavailability of drugs.
b. Describe the objectives of hospital pharmacy.
c. Describe the various methods of procurement of medicaments in hospital.

Q 3. Write short notes on (any *three*):

a. Teratogenicity
b. General treatment of poisoning
c. Drug information service
d. Location of hospital pharmacy
e. Pharmaceutical counselling

Q 4. What do you know about (any *three)*:

a. Constitution of pharmacy and therapeutic committee
b. Evaluation of absorbent cotton
c. Nonsterile manufacture
d. Out-patient services

Q 5.

a. Describe the symptoms and pathophysiology of tuberculosis or hepatitis.
b. How computers are useful in maintenance of records.

Or

Draw the layout of an ideal hospital and explain importance of ideal hospital.

Q 6. Attempt any *four* of the following:

a. What are the reasons for drug-abuse? How drug addicts are treated.
b. What is acute-poisoning? How lead poisoning is treated?
c. Explain with suitable examples, drug induced dermatological reactions.
d. What advice a pharmacist should offer to the patient in the treatment with the following drugs, any two:
   i. Castrol oil
   ii. Antacid tablets
   iii. Oxyphenbutazone
e. Explain the requirements and abilities required for pharmacists.
f. How the floor area and number of pharmacists required in an hospital pharmacy, are worked out?

Summer Examination 2000

D Pharm Second Year

Hospital and Clinical Pharmacy

Q 1.

a. Define any *five* of the following:

i. Hospital
ii. Clinical pharmacy
iii. Nonsterile manufacture
iv. Drug-abuse
v. Bioavailability of drugs
vi. Pre-packaging
vii. Economic order quantity

b. What you know about (any *two*):

i. Drug information centre
ii. Teratogenicity
iii. Drug interaction

Q 2. Write short notes on (any *two*):

a. Pharmacy and therapeutics committee
b. Hospital formulary system
c. Computers in maintenance of pharmacy

Q 3. Answer any *three* of the following:

a. State the importance of patient counselling.
b. Narrate the importance of physiological parameters in diagnosis of diseases.
c. Symptoms and pathophysiology of diabetes.
d. Describe symptoms and treatment of arsenic-poisoning.

Q 4. Attempt any *three* of the following:

a. Describe the technical and administrative abilities required by a pharmacist.
b. What you know about the containers and closures used in the parenterals?
c. Name various methods of sterilisation along with their merits and demerits.
d. What are the quality requirements of water for injection?

Q 5. Solve any *three* of the following:

a. Describe the evaluation and tests for identity of absorbent cotton.
b. What is purchase order? How it is prepared and state to whom the copies are distributed.
c. What are unpredictable adverse drug reactions? How they are classified?
d. Explain four mechanisms of drug interaction.

Q 6. Write short notes on (any *three*):

a. Universal antidote, in the treatment of poisoning.
b. Psychologic drug dependence.
c. Pharmaceutical factors affecting the bioavailability of drugs.
d. HEPA filters.

Winter Examination 2000

D Pharm Second Year

Hospital and Clinical Pharmacy

Q 1. Attempt the following:

a. Answer (any *two*):
   i. What do you mean by analgesics and antipyretics.

ii. What is patient counseling?
iii. What is clinical pharmacy?

b. Define (any *two*):
i. Hospital pharmacy
ii. Unit-dose dispensing
iii. Bioavailability of drugs

c. Explain the formation terms (any *four*):
i. Emetics
ii. Astringents
iii. Analeptics
iv. Tranquilizers
v. Cholagogue
vi. Purgatives

d. What advice must be given to the patients using (any *four*):
i. Salicylate
ii. Sulfa drugs
iii. Diazepam
iv. Chloramphenicol
v. Phenolphthalein
vi. Ampicillin

e. Translate into English (any *four*):
i. Pulvis
ii. Dandus
iii. Ana
iv. Semel
v. Secundus
vi. Cataplasma

Q 2. Attempt any *two* of the following:

a. Describe in short the processing involved in sterile manufacture.
b. Explain the process of dispensing drugs to out-patients in a typical hospital.
c. Describe the symptoms and pathophysiology of peptic ulcer.

Q 3. Answer any *four* of the following:

a. What are surgical dressings? Name the various pharmacopoeial tests to be performed on absorbent cotton wool IP.
b. State the functions of pharmacy and therapeutic committee.
c. Describe the objectives of a hospital pharmacy service.
d. What are physiological parameters? Explain their use with two suitable examples.
e. State the signs and symptoms of rhumatoid arthritis.
f. Who is administrator of a hospital? What are his responsibilities?

Q 4. Attempt any *four* of the following:

a. What is bed-side pharmacy?Give its importance.
b. Define and classify adverse drug reactions.
c. What are surgical instruments? Name any three with uses.
d. Give short account of hospital classified on the basis of ownership.
e. Describe various requirements to manufacture tablets in an hospital.
f. Give conditions to be fulfilled by all parenteral preparations.

Q 5. Answer any *four* of the following:

a. What is tuberculosis? Mention drugs used to control or treat tuberculosis.
b. What is purchase requisition? To when it is sent for procurement.
c. Explain the use of computers in inventory control in a drug store.
d. Give classification of poisons with suitable examples.
e. Write a note on health delivery system in India.
f. What are the sources of collection of information.

Q 6. Attempt any *three* of the following:

a. What do you mean by centralised or decentralised purchases? Describe to whom the copies of purchase orders are given.
b. Give the general procedure for the production of syrups.
c. Write a note on abilities of a pharmacist.
d. Describe the manufacturing of large and small volume parenterals.

Summer Examination 2001

D Pharm Second Year

Hospital and Clinical Pharmacy

Q 1. Attempt the following:

a. Translate into English (any *four*):

i. Charta
ii. Haustous
iii. Nebula
iv. Nocte
v. Dandus
vi. Auristille

b. Define the following terms (any *four*):

i. Snuffs
ii. Poultices
iii. Tinctures
iv. Emulsions
v. Syrups
vi. Suppositories

c. Answer any *two* of the following:

i. What is drug information bulletin?
ii. Name two preservatives used in injection.
iii. What is bed-side pharmcy?

d. Define (any *two*):

i. Hospital pharmacy
ii. Immunity
iii. Drug-dependance

e. Mention the suitable method of sterilisation of the following with reason to prefer the method (any *two*):

i. Eye ointments
ii. Plastic containers used for IV infusions
iii. Surgical gloves

Q 2. Answer any *two* of the following:

a. Describe in short, how drugs are distributed to in-patients in a typical hospital?
b. What is drug addiction? Name three drugs which cause addiction. How it is treated?
c. Describe the conditions to be fulfilled by all parenteral preparations.

Q 3. Answer any *three* of the following:

a. Explain the narcotic drugs with their advantage and disadvantage.
b. What is pharmacy and therapeutic committee? State its functions.
c. What is unit-dose dispensing? Give the benefits of unit-dose dispensing.
d. Describe the signs and symptoms of hepatitis.
e. Describe in short the processing involved in sterile manufacture.

Q 4. Answer any *four* of the following:

a. Explain the significance of hospital formulary system.
b. Define and classify hospitals.
c. Write a note on tetragenicity.
d. What are poisons? Describe the steps involved in the treatment of poisoning.
e. What is clinical pharmacy? State its importance in short.
f. What are the responsibilities of administrator of a hospital?

Q 5. Solve any *four* of the following:

a. Define bioavailability and name factors affecting it.
b. How dispensing of charged nonfloor stock is carried out?
c. Draw a floor plan of sterile product area.
d. Differentiate between pysiological and physical drug dependance.
e. What do you mean by centralised or decentralised purchases? Describe to whom the purchase order is given.
f. Explain the pathophysiology of diabetes.

Q 6. Attempt any *four* of the following:

a. What is food-drug interaction? Explain with example.
b. Give the composition of universal antidote and mention its uses.
c. Give the applications of computer in maintenance of record in hospitals.
d. Write a note on health delivery system in India.
e. Give the uses of following:
   i. Glucometer
   ii. ECG machine
   iii. Laminar flow
f. Write a note on importance of DLC.

Winter Examination 2001

D Pharm Second Year

Hospital and Clinical Pharmacy

Q 1.

a. Define any *five* of the following:

i. Hospital
ii. Bioavailability
iii. Pharmacy and therapeutics committee
iv. Drug abuse
v. Patient compliance
vi. Drug inventory

b. Give the meanings of (any *five*):

i. DIB
ii. SVP
iii. Airlock
iv. Dyspnoea
v. Arrhythmia
vi. Necrosis

Q 2. Answe any *three* of the following:

a. What are the functions of a modern hospital?
b. Give the layout of a hospital pharmacy which also manufactures parenterals.
c. What service does the pharmacist give to out-patients?
d. What is a bulk concentrate?
e. Write a note on "central sterile services".

Q 3. Answer any *three* of the following:

a. What are BG set and IV set?
b. Discuss the role of clinical pharmacist.
c. What are the sources of information for DIS?
d. Describe the nature of the hospital formulary.
e. Give advantages and disadvantages of "floorstock drug distribution system".

Q 4. Answer any *three* of the following:

a. What is the advantage of the computer regarding drug information service?
b. Explain the biological factors that control bioavailability.
c. What is meant by a satellite pharmacy?
d. What are the types of hypodermic syringes? How are nondisposable syringes treated before reuse?
e. Write a note on "pharmacy and therapeutics committee".

Q 5. Answer any *three* of the following:

a. What are the benefits of patient counselling?
b. Explain the pathophysiology of tuberculosis.
c. Explain angina pectoris along with its signs and symptoms.
d. What is the significance of CSF chlorides and CSF glucose?

Q 6. Answer any *three* of the following:

a. What is meant by pharmacokinetic drug interaction?
b. What happens to a patient prescribed warfarin if he also takes tetracycline?
c. What is idiosyncrasy?
d. Classify poisonous substances.
e. Discuss the role of pharmacist in preventing "adverse drug reactions".

Summer Examination 2002

D Pharm Second Year

Hospital and Clinical Pharmacy

Q 1. Answer the following:

a. What advise must be given to the patient using (any *four*)?
   i. Diazepam
   ii. Boric acid
   iii. Sulfa drugs
   iv. Ampicillin
   v. Salicylate
   vi. Phenolphthalein
b. Give normal values of (any *four*):
   i. Cholesterol
   ii. Respiration rate
   iii. ESR
   iv. Pulse rate
   v. WBC count
   vi. Specific gravity of urine
c. Differentiate between drug addiction and drug habituation.
d. Define the following terms (any *four*):
   i. Drug-dependance
   ii. Sterilisation
   iii. Emulsion
   iv. Tablets
   v. Immunity
   vi. Tinctures

e. Attempt any *two* of the following:
   i. Who is an out-patient?
   ii. What is drug information bulletin?
   iii. What is laminar flow?

Q 2. Attempt any *four* of the following:

a. Name three surgical instruments with their uses.
b. Define the term bioavailability and name various factors affecting it.
c. Classify poisons with examples.
d. How dispensing of charged non-floor stock is carried out?
e. Give the composition of universal antidote and mention its uses.
f. Give benefits of unit dose drug distribution system.

Q 3. Answer any *three* of the following:

a. Name various standards prescribed by IP for purity of absorbent cotton.
b. Define clinical pharmacy and describe its scope.
c. Describe signs and symptoms of tuberculosis.
d. What is food-drug interaction? Explain with example.
e. Describe the abilities required of a hospital phrmacist.

Q 4. Solve any *three* of the following:

a. Draw floor plan of sterile product area.
b. Define hospitals and classify them with suitable examples.
c. Differentiate acute and chronic poisoning.
d. What is bed-side pharmacy? Give its importance.
e. Write a note on “drug information centre”.

Q 5. Answer any *four* of the following:

a. What is purchase requisition? To whom it is sent for procurement.
b. Give short account of the functions of hospitals.
c. Define hospital formulary and give its significance.
d. Give the methods of estimating demand of hospitals.
e. Write a short note on hallucinogens.
f. Describe the objectives of hospital pharmacy services.

Q 6. Solve any *three* of the following:

a. Name the types of glass used to prepare container. Explain principle involved in hydrolytic resistance test for glass.
b. Give the composition and function of pharmacy and therapeutic committee.
c. Give the application of computer in maintenance of records in hospitals.

d. Give the symptoms and pathophysiology of diabetes.
e. Describe pharmacokinetic drug interactions with examples.

Winter Examination 2002

D Pharm Second Year

Hospital and Clinical Pharmacy

Q 1. Answer the following:

a. Attemt (any *two*):
   i. What is unit dose dispensing?
   ii. What is clinical pharmacy?
   iii. Name two preservatives used in injection.

b. Translate into English (any *four*):
   i. Cataplasma
   ii. Ungentum
   iii. Unus
   iv. Trochiscus
   v. Semel
   vi. Succus

c. Give normal values and significance of (any *two*):
   i. Blood sugar
   ii. Haemoglobin
   iii. ESR

d. Explain the following terms (any *four*):
   i. Emetics
   ii. Immunity
   iii. Tranquilizers
   iv. Analeptics
   v. Drug-dependance
   vi. Clinic

e. Answer (any *two*):
   i. What are demulcents and expectorants?
   ii. What is laminar flow?
   iii. What are OTC products?

Q 2. Attempt any *three* of the following:

a. Define and classify hospitals.
b. What is manufacture of drugs? Name the equipments for manufacture of tablets.
c. Give various administrative patterns of central services.
d. Name different drug distribution systems in hospitals and define emergency out-patients and in-patients.
e. Give the objectives and scope of clinical pharmacy.

Q 3. Attempt any *three* of the following:

a. What are the various additive used in the preparation of parenteral products?

b. Describe the evaluation and tests for identity of absorbent cotton.
c. State the various reasons of adverse drug reactions. How are they prevented?
d. What are surgical dressings? Give its uses.
e. "Modern hospitals are community health centres". Explain the statement.

Q 4. Attempt any *three* of the following:

a. How dispensing of charged non-floor stock is carried out?
b. Write a note on teratogenicity.
c. Describe the symptoms and pathophysiology of peptic ulcer.
d. What is PTC? State its composition and functions.
e. Write a note on "medication errors".

Q 5. Attempt any *two* of the following:

a. Name the pharmaceutical factors which affect the bioavailability of drugs. Discuss any three factors.
b. What is drug addiction? Name three drugs which cause addiction. How it is treated?
c. What do you mean by centralised or decentralised purchages? Describe to whom the copies of purchage orders are given and why?

Q 6. Attempt any *three* of the following:

a. What are physiological parameters? Do they help in diagnosis of diseases? Explain with two suitable examples.
b. Write a note on health delivery system in India.
c. Who is administrator of a hospital? What are his responsibilities?
d. What are drug interactions? Explain the role of pharmacist in identifying and preventing drug interactions.
e. Write a note on "drug information centre".

Summer Examination 2003

D Pharm Second Year

Hospital and Clinical Pharmacy

Q 1.

a. Define any *five* of the following:

i. Hospital pharmacy
ii. Adverse drug reaction
iii. Patient compliance
iv. Drug dependance
v. Poison
vi. CSSD
vii. Clinical pharmacy

b. Give the meaning of any *five* of the following:

i. Positive pressure
ii. Floor stock
iii. Coma
iv. Anorexia
v. Flatulence
vi. Health delivery system

Q 2. Answer any *three* of the following:

a. Classify hospitals according to ownership.
b. Where should the hospital pharmacy be located?
c. What is meant by unit dose dispensing?
d. What are the facilities and equipment required for manufacture of liquid orals?
e. Write a note on patient counseling.

Q 3. Answer any *three* of the following:

a. Explain what is a Ryle's tube and catheter.
b. What are the tests for absorbent cotton according to IP?
c. Write a note on drug information centre.
d. Name two health accessories and their uses.
e. Write a note on "hospital formulary".

Q 4. Answer any *three* of the following:

a. How does the computer help regarding medication monitoring?
b. What are the abilities required of a hospital pharmacist?
c. What are the factors that determine manufacture of drugs within the hospital pharmacy?
d. What is surgical gauze? Give its uses.
e. Explain the symptoms and treatment for "heavy metal poisoning".

Q 5. Answer any *three* of the following:

a. What advise will you give to a patient taking oxyphenbutazone?
b. What are the disease manifestations due to hepatitis?
c. What is the significance of insulin deficiency?
d. What is the significance of ESR?
e. Write a note on "inventory control" in hospital pharmacy.

Q 6. Answer any *three* of the following:

a. What is meant by pharmacodynamic drug interactions? Give examples.
b. What happens to a patient prescribed tolbutamide and insulin injection when he takes aspirin also?
c. Explain teratogenicity.
d. What is bioavailability? How are drugs absorbed from GIT?
e. Explain the need and functions of PTC.

Winter Examination 2003

D Pharm Second Year

Hospital and Clinical Pharmacy

Q 1.

a. Define any *five* of the following:

i. Hospital
ii. Hospital pharmacy
iii. Out-patient
iv. Drug dependance
v. Hospital formulary
vi. Surgical dressing
vii. Drug addiction

b. Answer any *five* of the following:

i. Give the normal values of (any *two*):
1. Normal blood sugar level
2. Normal pulse rate in adults
3. Normal ESR level
4. Normal specific gravity of urine

ii. Answer (any *two*): What advise is given to patients prescribed.
1. Mctronidazolc
2. Salicylates
3. Ampicillin
4. Diphenhydramine

iii. Answer (any *two*): What are the following toxicities?
1. Ocular toxicity due to corticosteroids
2. Gastrointestinal toxicity due to NSAID's.
3. Ototoxicity due to streptomycin.
4. Haematological toxicity due to aspirin.

iv. Answer (any *two*): What is the use of the following?
1. Ryle's tube
2. Hemostatic forcep
3. Aspirating needle
4. Rectal syringes

v. Give the meaning of (any *two*):
1. Placebo
2. Amnesia
3. Flatulence
4. Osteoporosis

vi. Answer (any *two*): What happens to a patient prescribed?
1. Procainamide and sulphonamide
2. Reserpine and atropine
3. Tetracycline with consumption of milk
4. MAO inhibitors and cheese

vii. Answer (any *two*): What is the antidote for?
1. Ammonia gas inhalation poisoning
2. Arsenic poisoning
3. Barbiturate poisoning
4. Charas poisoning

Q 2. Answer any *three* of the following:

a. What is scope of clinical pharmacy?
b. Explain pathophysiology of tuberculosis.
c. Classify cardiovascular diseases with their manifestations.
d. What are advantages of patient counselling?
e. What is the significance of patient history.

Q 3. Answer any *three* of the following:

a. What are advantages and disadvantages of liquid orals?
b. Draw layout of sterile manufacturing area.

Summer Examination 2004

D Pharm Second Year

Hospital and Clinical Pharmacy

Q 1. Answer the following:

a. Translate into English (any *five*):
   i. Charta
   ii. Nebula
   iii. Mane
   iv. Unus
   v. Nocte
   vi. Guttae
   vii. Ana
   viii. Haustous
b. Define the following terms (any *five*):
   i. Snuffs
   ii. Poultices
   iii. Tinctures
   iv. Emulsions
   v. Suppositories
   vi. Tablets
   vii. Immunity
   viii. Drug abuse
c. What advice must be given to the patient using (any *five*):
   i. Haematinics
   ii. Boric acid
   iii. Vaginal contraceptive suppositories
   iv. Ampicillin
   v. Diazepam
   vi. Salicylates

vii. Sulfa drugs
viii. Phenolphthalein

d. Give the meaning of (any *five*):

i. Necrosis
ii. Coma
iii. Air lock
iv. DIB
v. Anorexia
vi. Insomnia
vii. Dyspnea
viii. Arrhythmia

Q 2. Attempt any *three* of the following:

a. Give the benefits of unit dose distribution system.
b. Define and classify hospitals.
c. What are surgical dressings? Give its uses.
d. Differentiate acute and chronic poisoning.
e. What is bed-side pharmacy? Give its importance.

Q 3. Attempt any *three* of the following:

a. What is hospital formulary? Give its importance.
b. Describe pharmacokinetic drug interactions with examples.
c. Draw floor plan of sterile product area.
d. Describe signs and symptoms of tuberculosis.
e. Give methods of estimating demand of hospital.

Q 4. Attempt any *three* of the following:

a. Define clinical pharmacy and describe its scope.
b. Give short account of hospital classified on the basis of ownership.
c. Write a note on health delivery system in India.
d. What are the functions of modern hospitals?
e. What is PTC? State its composition and functions.

Q 5. Attempt any *three* of the following:

a. Give the application of computer in maintenance of record in hospitals.
b. What is bulk concentrate?
c. Explain what is BT set and IV set.
d. Who is the administrator of a hospital? What are his responsibilities?
e. Write a note on satellite pharmacy?

Q 6. Attempt any *three* of the following:

a. Explain the biological factors that control bioavailability.
b. Give the composition of universal antidote and mention its use.
c. What are surgical instruments? Name any three with uses.
d. Write a note on importance of DLC.
e. Describe in short, how drugs are distributed to in-patients in a typical hospital.

Winter Examination 2004

D Pharm Second Year

Hospital and Clinical Pharmacy

Q 1.

a. Define any *five* of the following:

i. Out-patient
ii. Clinical pharmacy
iii. Bioavailability
iv. Hospital
v. Unit dose dispensing
vi. Drug abuse
vii. Patient counselling

b. Give the meaning of any *five* of the following:

i. Hallucinogen
ii. Teratogenicity
iii. Superinfection
iv. Contraindication
v. Hospital formulas
vi. Rate contract
vii. Pharmacy and therapeutic committee

Q 2. Attempt any *three* of the following:

a. Define hospital pharmacy. Give the objectives of hospital pharmacy.
b. How will you justify the role of pharmacist in management of central service? Comment on manpower requirements and location in sterile area.
c. Explain the stepwise procedure adopted for centralised purchase in hospital. Define reorder quantity.
d. Name any four surgical dressings. Give the standards for absorbant cotton.
e. What is rheumatoid arthritis? Comment on pathophysiology, signs and symptoms of rheumatoid arthritis.

Q 3. Attempt any *three* of the following:

a. i. What is the role of pharmacist in adverse drug reaction monitoring?
   ii. Comment on health delivery system in India on state and District level.
b. Explain the factors influencing make on buy decision in hospital. Name the methods of estimation of demand.
c. Name any four surgical instruments alongwith their uses.
d. Explain the role of computers in:
   i. Medication monitoring in hospital.
   ii. Purchasing and inventory control in hospital.

e. Give normal count and significance of following physiological parameters:
   i. Haemoglobin
   ii. ESR
   iii. Sperm count
   iv. Cholesterol

Q 4. Attempt any *three* of the following:

a. Give the requirements of location and layout of out-patient pharmacy.
b. Name various steps involved in manufacturing of sterile product. Explain filling operation in short.
c. Give the functions of pharmacy and therapeutic committee.
d. Define drug interaction. Give various mechanisms of drug interactions with one example of each.
e. Enumerate factors affecting bioavailability of drugs. What is bioequivalence?

Q 5. Attempt any *three* of the following:

a. What do you mean by floor stock system? Give the criteria for selection of charge floor stock drug. How they are dispensed?
b. What are the contents of hospital formulary? Comment on role of pharmacy and therapeutic committee in preparation of formulary.
c. Define patient compliance. Explain how patient counselling by pharmacist helps to improve patient compliance.
d. Classify adverse drug reactions. What are the probable causes of adverse drug reactions?
e. What is general line of treatment for drug abuse? Write a note on medical complications, withdrawal symptoms and treatment of alcoholism.

Q 6. Attempt any *three* of the following:

a. Give any four functions of a modern hospital. Classify hospital on the basis of ownership.
b. Name the equipments required for manufacturing of compressed tablets and pills.
c. How will you justify that pharmacist is suitable person to run drug information service? Comment on sources of information for drug information service.
d. What do you mean by drug induced diseases? Give various drug induced diseases.
e. Classify poisons. What are the steps involved in general treatment of poisoning?

Summer Examination 2005

D Pharm Second Year

Hospital and Clinical Pharmacy

Q 1. Attempt the following:

a. Answer the following (any *two*):
   i. Mention the use of BAL and EDTA in toxicology.
   ii. What is laminar air flow?
   iii. What is drug information service?

b. What advice must be given to the patient using (any *four*):
   i. Boric acid
   ii. Diazepam
   iii. Ampicillin
   iv. Phenytoin
   v. Bisacodyl
   vi. MAO inhibitors

c. Give normal values and significance of (any *two*):
   i. RBC count
   ii. ESR
   iii. Clotting time of blood

d. Translate into English (any *four*):
   i. Dandus
   ii. Semel in die
   iii. Unus
   iv. Tussis
   v. Unguentem
   vi. Nuristillae

e. Explain the following (any *two*):
   i. IV set
   ii. Rubber catheter
   iii. ECG machine
   iv. CT scanner

Q 2. Answer any *three* of the following:

a. Define and classify hospitals.
b. What are the functions of hospital pharmacy? Describe technical abilities required for a hospital pharmacist.
c. Define nonsterile manufacturing of drugs. What are equipments required for liquid orals?
d. Describe objectives of hospital pharmacy.
e. What is role of nursing department in a hospital?

Q 3. Answer any *three* of the following:

a. Discuss about location and layout of OPD.
b. What is clinical pharmacy? Describe its scope.
c. Define unit dose dispensing. How dispensing of non-charge floor stock drug is carried out?
d. Explain pathophysiology of epilepsy.
e. Write short notes on (any *two*):
   i. Idiosyncrasy
   ii. Drug dependence

Q 4. Answer any *three* of the following:

a. What are drug interaction? Explain two mechanisms of pharmacodynamic interaction.
b. Define ADR. Give causes of ADR.
c. Give three administrative patterns of central sterile service.
d. Give the composition of pharmacy and therapeutic committee. Write in short role of PTC in a drug safety.
e. Define the term hospital formulary. Write guiding principles while using a formulary.

Q 5. Answer any *three* of the following:

a. What are gauze and bandages? Name the various pharmacopoeial tests for absorbent cotton wool.
b. Give any three drugs which are drugs of addiction. How drug abuse is treated?
c. Name the various subdivisions of sterile product area. What are various additives in the parenteral?
d. Describe the procedure for procurement of materials in hospital.
e. What is bedside and satellite pharmacy?

Q 6. Answer any *three* of the following:

a. How does the computer help regarding medication monitoring?
b. Classify poisons in short. How narcotic-drugs poisoning is treated?
c. What is bioequivalence? Discuss three physiological factors which affect the bioavailability of drugs.
d. Describe signs and symptoms of rheumatoid arthritis.
e. What are the economic considerations which govern the decisions to make or buy drugs in hospital pharmacy?

Winter Examination 2005
D Pharm Second Year
Hospital and Clinical Pharmacy

Q 1. Answer the following:

a. **Attempt (any *two*):**
   i. Write a short note on additives in parenterals.
   ii. What is hospital pharmacy?
   iii. What is bed-side pharmacy services?

b. **Define (any *two*):**
   i. Patient compliance
   ii. Bioavailability of drugs
   iii. Universal antidote

c. **Explain the following terms (any *four*):**
   i. Anti-sialagogues
   ii. Bitters
   iii. Achlorhydria
   iv. Cholagogue
   v. Tincture
   vi. Tranquilizers

d. **What advice must be given to the patient using (any *four*)**
   i. Antacid tablet
   ii. Liquid paraffin
   iii. Penicillins
   iv. Tetracycline
   v. Salicylate
   vi. Nitrates

e. **Give the meaning of the following Latin terms (any *four*):**
   i. Unguentum
   ii. Nebula
   iii. Radix
   iv. Mistura

Q 2. Attempt any *two* of the following:

a. Describe the qualifications and abilities required of hospital pharmacist.
b. Describe the symptoms and pathophysiology of *angina pectoris*.
c. Write a note on central sterile services.

Q 3. Answer any *four* of the following:

a. State the function of pharmacy and therapeutic committee.
b. Define and classify adverse drug reactions.
c. Write a short note on health delivery system in India.
d. Write a short note on location and layout of OPD.
e. Describe two factors affecting make or buy decision in hospital.
f. Describe the layout of sterile product area.

Q 4. Attempt any *four* of the following:

a. Explain the role of pharmacist in patient counselling.
b. What are surgical instruments? Name any four with uses.
c. Define bandage and classify with examples.
d. What is clinical pharmacy? Give its scope.
e. What are the objectives of hospital formulary system?
f. Explain the different sources of drug information.

Q 5. Attempt any *three* of the following:

a. What is non-sterile manufacturing? Give method of production of syrup.
b. Give the objectives of purchasing and inventory control.
c. Describe the use of computer in maintenance of record.
d. What is diabetes mellitus and give its types.
e. Give the clinical significance of the following:
   i. Blood pressure
   ii. Blood cholesterol
   iii. ESR
   iv. Blood sugar level

Q 6. Attempt any *three* of the following:

a. Define "hospital" and classify hospital on the basis of clinical orientation.
b. Define drug interaction and classify the mechanism of drug interaction.
c. Differentiate between drug addiction and drug habituation.
d. Define drug dependence and explain its different types.
e. What is acute poisoning? Write treatment of arsenic poisoning.

Summer Examination 2006
D Pharm Second Year
Hospital and Clinical Pharmacy

Q 1. Solve any *five* of the following:

a. Write the normal range of:
   i. MCV — iii. ALP
   ii. AST — iv. ALT
b. Define the following terms:
   i. Etiology — ii. Ostomy
c. State the meaning of:
   i. Carminatives — iii. Anorexia
   ii. Emetics — iv. Dyspnea
d. Write the antidotes for:
   i. Physostigmine — iii. Ethylene glycol
   ii. Pentazocine — iv. Quinidine
e. State the meaning of:
   i. Bioequivalence — ii. Lithotripsy
f. Define the following:
   i. Immunity and susceptibility
   ii. Antagonism and synergism
g. Write one example of each of the following poisons:
   i. Corrosives — iii. Organic
   ii. Irritants — iv. Inorganic

Q 2. Solve any *three* of the following:

a. Discuss the health delivery system in India.
b. Classify different types of ADR with examples.
c. Discuss the terms—General patient, Referred patient, Emergency patient, Ambulatory patient.
d. Discuss the different LFT parameters of clinical significance with their normal range.

e. Write the normal values for:
   i. Hb in adult male and female
   ii. RBC in adult male and female

Q 3. Solve any *three* of the following:

a. Discuss the measurement of bioavailability.
b. Discuss the official sterility test for evaluation of parenterals.
c. Name various methods of sterilisation. Write the principle involed in autoclaving.
d. Classify leucocytes. Write its characteristics and normal count.
e. Discuss the floor stock system with its merits and demerits.

Q 4. Solve any *three* of the following:

a. Give the composition and functions of PTC.
b. Write the teratogenic effects of:
   i. Thalidomide ii. Diethylstilbesterol
c. Discuss the professional requirements for the chief hospital pharmacist.
d. Comment on pathophysiology, signs and symptoms of myocardial infarction.
e. State the meaning of patient compliance and discuss the different types of noncompliance and its consequences.

Q 5. Solve any *three* of the following:

a. Describe hospitals on the basis of ownership.
b. Discuss how BAL is effective as an antidote for arsenic poisoning and discuss its dose and schedule of administration.
c. Discuss the role, significance and the guiding principles of hospital formulary system.
d. What is CSD? Give objectives and the working of CSD in hospital organisation.
e. State the meaning of following:
   i. Icterus iii. Hodgkin's disease
   ii. Addison's disease iv. Buerger's disease

Q 6. Solve any *three* of the following:

a. State eight functions of hospital pharmacy.
b. Discuss drug interaction mechanisms considering pharmacodynamic factors.
c. What are antidotes? Classify different types of antidotes with examples.
d. What are the withdrawal symptoms of alcohol and write treatment for it.
e. Discuss the use of computer in pharmacy.

Winter Examination 2006

D Pharm Second Year

Hospital and Clinical Pharmacy

Q 1. Answer the following:

a. Define (any *four*):

i. Drug addiction	iv. Elixirs
ii. Immunity	v. Tranquillisers
iii. Emulsion	vi. Anthelminthics

b. Explain the following (any *four*):

i. Etiology	iv. Purgatives
ii. Analeptics	v. Rate contract
iii. Emetics	vi. Astringents

c. Give normal values of (any *four*):

i. Pulse rate	iv. ESR
ii. Blood sugar	v. RBC count
iii. Specific gravity of urine	vi. Clotting time of blood

d. What advice must be given to the patients using (any *four*):

i. Antacid tablet	iv. Salicylates
ii. Diazepam	v. Ampicillin
iii. Sulfa drugs	vi. Bisacodyl

e. Translate into English (any *four*):

i. Collutorium	iv. Semel in die
ii. Nebula	v. Dolore urgente
iii. Cataplasma	vi. Folium

Q 2. Attempt any *three* of the following:

a. What is hospital formulary? Explain in short about entry and deletion of drug in the formulary.

b. Draw a layout of sterile manufacturing area.

c. Define surgical dressing. Describe two tests to evaluate absorbent cotton.

d. Define the term drug interaction. Describe at least three examples of drug-food interaction.

e. What are surgical instruments? Name any three with uses.

Q 3. Answer any *three* of the following:

a. What is pharmacy and therapeutic committee? State its functions.

b. Explain the method of dispensing drugs to out-patients in typical hospital.

c. Define clinical pharmacy and describe its scope.

d. Write a note on teratogenicity.

e. What is bioavailability of drugs? Discuss two pharmaceutical factors affecting bioavailability.

Q 4. Attempt any *three* of the following:

a. Describe patient counseling by pharmacist in short.
b. Give layout of an ideal hospital organization.
c. What are the functions of modern hospitals?
d. Write the symptoms and explain pathophysiology of peptic ulcer.
e. Define hospital pharmacy. State the objectives of hospital pharmacy.

Q 5. Answer any *three* of the following:

a. What is antidote? Give the composition of universal antidote.
b. Describe the application of computer in maintenance of record in hospitals.
c. Describe various requrements to undertake the manufacture of tablets in a hospital.
d. Write an account on hospital classified on the basis of ownership.
e. Describe the location and layout of central sterile service.

Q 6. Attempt any *three* of the following:

a. Give benefits of unit dose system.
b. State general procedure for production of syrup.
c. Write a note on laminar flow.
d. Explain two pharmacodynamics mechanisms of drug interaction.
e. Write a note on health delivery system in India.
f. Describe two abilities required for hospital pharmacist.

Summer Examination 2007

D Pharm Second Year

Hospital and Clinical Pharmacy

Q 1. Answer any *five* of the following:

a. Give the normal values of (any *two*):

i. Cholesterol	iii. Haemoglobin
ii. Blood sugar level	

b. Translate into English (any *four*):

i. Ungentum	iv. Haustous
ii. Nocte	v. Mane
iii. Trochiscus	vi. Folium

c. Explain the following terms (any *four*):

i. Analeptics	iv. Immunity
ii. Tinctures	v. Emetics
iii. Drug dependence	vi. Antibiotics

d. What advice must be given to the patients using (any *two*):

i. Phenolphthalein
ii. Haematinics
iii. Sulfa drugs
iv. Diazepam

e. Answer (any *two*):

i. Discuss the role of "clinical pharmacist".
ii. What is drug information bulletin?
iii. What are 'demulcents' and expectorants?

f. Give the meanings of (any *four*):

i. Airlock
ii. Necrosis
iii. SVP
iv. Dyspnea
v. Arrhythmia

Q 2. Attempt any *three* of the following:

a. What is PTC? Describe its role in drug safety.
b. Explain the process of dispensing drugs to out-patients in a typical hospital.
c. What is drug addiction? Name three drugs which cause addiction? How it is treated?
d. Define and classify hospitals.
e. Write a note on role of administrator in hospital organizations.

Q 3. Attempt any *three* of the following:

a. Give the general procedure for the production of syrups.
b. Describe various requirements to manufacture tablets in hospital.
c. Give conditions to be fulfilled by all parenteral preparations.
d. Define and classify adverse drug reactions.
e. Define the terms hospital pharmacy. Write functions of hospital pharmacy.

Q 4. Attempt any *three* of the following:

a. Explain the use of computers in inventory control in a drug store.
b. What is unit dose dispensing? Give the benefits of unit dose dispensing.
c. Give the composition of universal antidote and mention its uses.
d. Write a note on 'contents of hospital formulary'.
e. Define surgical dressing. Describe different types of bandages.

Q 5. Attempt any *three* of the following:

a. State the signs and symptoms of rheumatoid arthritis.
b. What are poisons? Describe the steps involved in the treatment of poisoning.
c. Explain the pathophysiology of diabetes mellitus.
d. What is central sterile service? Describe its layout.
e. Explain the pathophysiology of tuberculosis.

Q 6. Attempt any *three* of the following:

a. Write a note on patient counseling.
b. Mention various pharmaceutical factors affecting the bioavailability of drugs.
c. Explain four mechanisms of drug interaction.
d. Describe treatment of drug abuse.
e. What is idiosyncrasy?

Winter Examination 2007

D Pharm Second Year

Hospital and Clinical Pharmacy

Q 1. Answer the following questions:

a. Answer of the following (any *two*):
   i. Define bioavailability and list the various factors which affect bioavailability.
   ii. Who are the members of PTC? Give four functions which they need to perform.
   iii. Write primary and secondary sources of drug information bulletin.

b. Give normal values and significance of (any *two*):
   i. RBC count
   ii. Blood sugar
   iii. Prothrombin time

c. Translate into English (any *four*):
   i. Ter in die
   ii. Secundis horis
   iii. Parvus
   iv. Magnus
   v. Semis horis
   vi. Tincturae

d. What advice must be given to patients using (any *four*):
   i. Liquid paraffin
   ii. Boric acid
   iii. Phenyl butazone and oxyphen butazone
   iv. Antacid tablets
   v. Salicylates
   vi. Diphenhydramine

Q 2. Answer any *three* of the following:

a. Describe the objectives of hospital parmacy.
b. Write a note on location and layout of hospital pharmacy.
c. Define a modern hospital. Describe four major functions of a hospital.
d. Describe at least eight functions of a hospital administrator.

e. What is the purpose of medical records? What are the basic principles in preparing them?

Q 3. Answer any *three* of the following:

a. Describe the abilities required for a hospital pharmacist run the hospital pharmacy successfully.
b. What services are provided by pharmacist to out-patient?
c. What are the advantages of prepacking drugs?
d. Name two databases having medical and pharmaceutical literature. What do you know about drug information retrieval?
e. What are adverse drug reactions? Classify the types. How are they be reduced?

Q 4. Answer any *three* of the following:

a. With examples mention drug induced renal diseases.
b. Explain the concept of clinical pharmacy. State the objectives of clinical pharmacy.
c. What is patient compliance? Explain the reasons for non-compliance? What is the phrmacists role in improving compliance?
d. Name the different types of forceps used in hospitals (draw their diagram). How are they sterilized?
e. Which are the different items purchased in the stores of hospital? When is it decided to place the order for more materials?

Q 5. Answer any *three* of the following:

a. What is UDDS? Write advantages and disadvantages of this system.
b. What is hospital formulary? Write its significance.
c. What care should the personnel working in sterile department take for working in aseptic area.
d. What are the official evaluation tests for parenterals? Write a note on pyrogen testing.
e. Classify poisons. How is the general treatment for poisoning is done?

Q 6. Answer any *three* of the following:

a. Classify pharmacokinetic drug interactions. With examples explain the drug interactions related to distribution alteration.
b. Explain the terms drug abuse and drug habituation. How is the treatment of drug abuse done?
c. What are the signs and symptoms of duodenal ulcer?
d. Write a note on teratogenicity.
e. Classify the hospitals on clinical basis.

Summer Examination 2008

D Pharm Second Year

Hospital and Clinical Pharmacy

Q 1. Attempt the following:

a. Define the following (any *four*):
   - i. DIC
   - ii. Clinical pharmacy
   - iii. Teratogenicity
   - iv. Bioavailability
   - v. Physiological parameters
   - vi. Patient compliance

b. Give normal values and significance of following (any *two*):
   - i. Haemoglobin
   - ii. RBC
   - iii. Blood sugar

c. What advice must be given to the patient using (any *four*):
   - i. Chloramphenicol
   - ii. Boric acid
   - iii. MAO inhibitor
   - iv. Phenolphthalein
   - v. Ampicillin
   - vi. Diphenhydramine

d. Mention the use of following (any *four*):
   - i. Laminar air flow
   - ii. CT scanner
   - iii. MRI
   - iv. Lithotripsy
   - v. ECG
   - vi. Haemostatic forcep

e. Translate into English (any *two*):
   - i. SOS
   - ii. Omnihora
   - iii. Charta

f. Explain following term (any *two*):
   - i. Presbyopia
   - ii. Stenosis
   - iii. Sialogogue

Q 2. Attempt any *three* of the following:

a. What is decentralized purchase. Write procedure adopted by hospital pharmacist to procure drugs or hospital supplies.

b. Give various administrative pattern of CSSR.

c. What is the purpose of medical record? Give its contents.

d. Explain dispensing of non-charge floor stock drugs in hospital.

e. Discuss economic factors governing the make or buy decision.

Q 3. Attempt any *three* of the following:

a. Write a note on:
   - i. Allergy
   - ii. Anaphylaxis

b. Define drug interaction. Explain what happens when:
   - i. Cathartics are given with sustained released drugs.
   - ii. Folic acid is given along with phenytoin.

c. What is bed side pharmacy? Give its importance.
d. How surgical cotton is evaluated as per IP?
e. Define drug abuse. Give its general treatment.

Q 4. Attempt any *three* of the following:

a. Explain why kidney is highly sensitive to effects of drugs with examples.
b. Define out-patient. What services are provided to out-patient by pharmacist?
c. Define hallucinogen. Give effects and treatment of LSD.
d. How PTC ensures drug safety in hospital.
e. Differentiate between drug addiction and drug habituation.

Q 5. Attempt any *three* of the following:

a. Discuss physiological factors affecting bioavailability of drugs.
b. Classify poisons. Enlist steps involved in general treatment of poisoning.
c. What are the requirements of aseptic area? State precautions in aseptic area.
d. Write applications of computer in retail pharmacy.
e. Write a note on containers and closures used in parenterals.

Q 6. Attempt any *three* of the following:

a. Who is an administrator? What are his responsibilities?
b. What is tuberculosis? Write its pathophysiology, signs and symptoms.
c. Define and classify hospital on the basis of ownership.
d. What is hospital formulary? What are the requirements for preparation of HF?
e. What is chronic poisoning? Give signs and symptoms and treatment of narcotic poisoning?

Winter Examination 2008

D Pharm Second Year

Hospital and Clinical Pharmacy

Q 1. Attempt any *five* of the following:

a. Define the following terms:
   i. Bioequivalence
   ii. Adverse drug reaction
b. State the meaning of following (any *four*):
   i. Tranquilizer
   ii. Haematinics
   iii. Immunity
   iv. Carminative
   v. Anesthetics
   vi. Emetics

c. Mention the suitable method of sterilization for any *four* of the following:
   i. Rubber hand globes
   ii. Eye ointment
   iii. Intramuscular oily injection
   iv. Surgical dressings
   v. Normal saline for injection
   vi. Plastic containers for sterile solution

d. What advice should be given to a patient using:
   i. Tetracyclines
   ii. Vaginal contraceptive pessaries
   iii. Phenolphthalein
   iv. MAO inhibitors?

e. Define the following terms:
   i. Clinical pharmacy
   ii. Drug interaction

f. Give the normal values of (any *four*):
   i. RBC count
   ii. Blood cholesterol in young adults
   iii. Hb count in male
   iv. Eosinophils
   v. Sperm count
   vi. Fasting blood sugar

Q 2. Attempt any *three* of the following:

a. Define central services. Mention three administrative patterns of central service. Discuss how central service department is related with hospital pharmacist.

b. Discuss the factors governing make or buy decision in hospital.

c. Define hospital. How adminstrator plays a key role in hospital management.

d. What are the sources of information for drug information centre? Justify how pharmacist is better qualified to run drug information centre.

e. What is surgical cotton? How it is standardised as per Indian pharmacopoeia?

Q 3. Attempt any *three* of the following:

a. Discuss the health delivery systems in India.

b. Name the tests used for evaluation of parenterals in hospitals discuss pyrogen testing.

c. Define clinical pharmacy. Discuss six barriers for development of clinical pharmacy in India.

d. Classify adverse drug reaction and discuss any one from it.
e. What is drug dependence? Give medical complications withdrawal symptoms and treatment of alcoholism.

Q 4. Attempt any *three* of the following:

a. Discuss the pathophysiology, signs, symptoms and treatment of tuberculosis.
b. Write the eight function of pharmacy and therapeutic committee in hospital.
c. Define bioavailability and discuss the factors affecting bioavailability.
d. Define hospital pharmacy. Discuss the functions and objectives of hospital pharmacy.
e. What is difference between centralised and decentralised purchase? Define re-order quantity. Write a note on rate contract.

Q 5. Attempt any *three* of the following:

a. State the meaning of out-patient. Discuss location and layout of out-patient services in hospital.
b. Give an organization chart of a hospital pharmacy service. Discuss the abilities of a hospital pharmacist.
c. State the meaning of hospital formulary? Write six guiding principles while using hospital formulary.
d. i. Write the uses of following surgical instruments:
   1. Tissue forceps
   2. Scalpel
   3. Laminectomy saw
   4. Aneurysm needle

   ii. Discuss the drug food interation
e. What is diabetes mellitus? Discuss pathophysiology, signs and symptoms of diabetes mellitus.

Q 6. Attempt any *three* of the following:

a. Discuss how computers are useful in hospital for:
   i. Purchasing and inventory control
   ii. Medication monitoring
b. Define patient compliance and patient counseling. What are the various areas in which pharmacist can advice the patient?
c. Define unit dose dispensing. Give any three benefits of unit dose dispensing. Mention any four criteria for selection of non-charge floor stock drugs.
d. Classify poisons according to their mode of action. What are the steps involved in general treatment of poisoning?
e. Comment on pharmacokinetic interaction with examples.

Summer Examination 2009

D Pharm Second Year

Hospital and Clinical Pharmacy

Q 1. Attempt the following:

a. Define the following (any *four*):
   i. Drug dependence
   ii. Immunity
   iii. Suppository
   iv. Tranquilizers
   v. Patient compliance

b. Give normal values of (any *four*):
   i. Haemoglobin
   ii. Sperm count
   iii. Cholesterol
   iv. Clotting time, bleeding time of blood
   v. Blood sugar

c. What advice must be given to the patient using (any *four*):
   i. Phenolphthalein
   ii. Sulfa drug
   iii. Bisacodyl
   iv. Phenytoin
   v. Ampicillin

d. Translate into English (any *four*):
   i. Nuristillae
   ii. Haustas
   iii. Prn
   iv. Unguentum
   v. Dolore urgente

e. State the meaning of (any *four*):
   i. IVP
   ii. Lithotripsy
   iii. DIB
   iv. Flatulence
   v. Positive pressure

Q 2. Attempt any *three* of the following:

a. Define hospital. Classify hospital with examples.
b. Explain what is a 'Ryles tube' and 'Rubber catheter'?
c. What is unit dose dispensing? Give its benefits.
d. What are objectives of hospital pharmacy?
e. Discuss economic factors governing the manufacture or purchase decision in production.

Q 3. Answer any *three* of the following:

a. What is 'hospital formulary'? Give its contents.
b. Who is an administrator? What are his responsibilities?

c. Explain the use of computers in inventory control in a drug store.
d. What are surgical instruments? Name any three with their uses.
e. Describe the location and layout of central sterile service room.

Q 4. Attempt any *three* of the following:

a. Define clinical pharmacy and describe its scope.
b. Describe signs, symptoms and pathophysiology of 'diabetes'.
c. What is meant by pharmacodynamic drug interactions? Give examples.
d. Define ADR. Give causes of ADR.
e. What are poisons? Describe the steps involved in treatment of poison.

Q 5. Answer any *three* of the following:

a. Differentiate between 'drug addiction' and 'drug habituation'.
b. Explain physiological factors affecting bioavailability. What is bioequivalence?
c. What is the significance of patient history?
d. What are withdrawal symptoms of alcohol and write treatment for it?
e. What is:
   i. Idiosyncrasy ii. Allergy

Q 6. Attempt any *three* of the following:

a. What happens to a patient prescribed tolbutamide and insulin injection when he takes aspirin also?
b. How many purchase orders are prepared? To whom it can be sent?
c. Give conditions fullfill by the parenteral. Enlist the equipment needed for the preparation of parenterals.
d. What is 'out-patient'? Give its detail classification.
e. Give pathophysiology, signs and symptoms of 'rheumatoid arthritis'.

Summer Examination 2010
D Pharm Second Year
Hospital and Clinical Pharmacy

Q 1. Answer the following:

a. Define the following: (Any *two*)
   i. Unit dose dispensing
   ii. Out patient
   iii. Drug dependence

b. Mention antidote for following: (Any *four*)
   i. Arsenic
   ii. Iron
   iii. Capper
   iv. Lead
   v. Morphine
c. Write normal values with significance: (Any *two*)
   i. Blood cholesterol
   ii. Blood-sugar
   iii. Heart rate
d. Write the meaning of following: (Any *four*)
   i. Hematinics
   ii. Etiology
   iii. Analeptics
   iv. Purgatives
   v. Glycosuria
   vi. Pathogenesis
e. Answer the following: (Any *two*)
   i. What is counselling by pharmacist?
   ii. What are elite hospitals?
   iii. What advice is given by pharmacist when antidiabetic drug and diazepam is prescribed?

Q 2. Answer any *three* of the following:

a. Define hallucinogens. Write effects of LSD.
b. How dosage form affects bioavailability of drug?
c. Define hospital. What is the role of administrator in hospital?
d. When universal antidote is used? Give its composition.
e. Write sign, symptoms and treatment of acute arsenic poisoning.

Q 3. Answer *three* of the following:

a. What are teratogens? Give two examples of teratogenic drugs along with its teratogenic effects.
b. Define drug interaction and explain two example of food drug interaction.
c. Give reasons of adverse drug reactions.
d. Explain what happens when the following drugs are prescribed together:
   i. Warfarin and phenyl butazone
   ii. Digitalis and diuretic
e. Define DIB. Give its importance.

Q 4. Answer *three* of the following:

a. What is clinical pharmacy? Give its objectives.
b. Write pathophysiology and symptoms of atherosclerosis.
c. How computers are useful in maintenance of records?
d. Define bandages. How neps, acidity-alkalinity and surface active agent test is performed on cotton?
e. Explain uses of BAL and desferrioxamine in toxicology.

Q 5. Answer *three* of the following:

a. Write guidelines for entry and deletion of drugs in formulary.
b. Where should CSSR be located in hospital? How should be its layout?
c. Describe purchase procedure step by step.
d. What are the requirements of aseptic area?
e. Define PTC. Give its role in drug safety.

Q 6. Answer *three* of the following:

a. Name the test for evaluation of parenterals. Describe any one.
b. Define drug dependence. Explain its type.
c. Write four functions and four objectives of hospital pharmacy.
d. Mention the different drug distribution systems to in-patient. What is satellite pharmacy?
e. Give the uses of following: (Any *four*)
   i. CT scanner
   ii. Ultrasound sonography
   iii. Lithotripsy
   iv. X-ray machine
   v. ECG machine

Winter Examination 2010

D Pharm Second Year

Hospital and Clinical Pharmacy

Q 1. Attempt the following:

a. Define any two of the followings:
   i. Drug abuse
   ii. Hospital
   iii. Clinical pharmacy
   iv. ADR
b. State the meaning of any four:
   i. Emetics
   ii. Anorexia
   iii. PTC
   iv. Teretogenicity
   v. Purgative
   vi. Patient counselling
c. Give normal values of any four:
   i. Blood cholesterol
   ii. Blood sugar
   iii. Haemoglobin
   iv. ESR

v. Clotting time of blood
vi. Specific gravity of urine

d. Write one example of each of the following poison:
i. Corrosive
ii. Organic
iii. Inorganic
iv. Irritant

e. What advices must be given to the patient while using (any *four*)
i. Phenytoin
ii. Diazepam
iii. Sulphadrugs
iv. MAO-inhibitors
v. Antacid
vi. Ampicillin

Q 2. Attempt any *three*:

a. Name any four surgical dressings. Give the standards for absorbent cotton wool.
b. Name various methods of sterilization. Give principle of hot air oven and autoclave.
c. Discuss the "Health delivery system in India".
d. What is bio-equivalence? Discuss three physiological factors affect the bio-availability of drug.
e. Give the functions of PTC with their objectives.

Q 3. Attempt any *three*:

a. Name any four surgical instruments with their uses.
b. Classify ADR. Discuss its causes.
c. What do you mean by drug induced diseases? Give various such diseases.
d. What economical consideration will be taken to make or buy drugs in hospital? Name methods of estimation of demands.
e. Classify hospital on clinical and non-clinical basis.

Q 4. Attempt any *three*:

a. Define non-sterile manufacturing. What are requirements of equipment for compressed tablets and pills?
b. Define "Hospital pharmacist". Give different abilities a "Hospital pharmacist" should passes.
c. Draw a line-long out of "ideal modern hospital"
d. Give the administration pattern for hospitals.
e. Describe sign, symptoms and pathophysiology of peptic ulcer or rheumatoid arthritis.

Q 5. Attempt any *three*:

a. Give importance of "Nursing services" and "medical record services" in hospital.
b. Define "Unit dose drug distribution system". Write its benefits.
c. Name various subdivisions of sterile product area. What are various additives used in parenterals.
d. Discuss the term General patient, Referred patient, Emergency patient and Ambulatory patient.
e. What is patient compliance? Discuss various types of non-compliance and its consequences.

Q 6. Attempt any *three*:

a. What is hospital formulary? Give guideline principles for preparation of hospital formulary.
b. Explain how purchase order is prepared and distributed.
c. Give classification of poison. What are steps involve in general treatment of poisoning.
d. Define drug interaction. Give various mechanism of drug interaction with one example of each.
e. Explain the role of computer in purchasing and inventory control in hospital and medication history of patient.

Summer Examination 2011

D Pharm Second Year

Hospital and Clinical Pharmacy

Q 1. Answer the following questions:

a. Define any four:
   i. Drug interaction
   ii. Pyrogens
   iii. Unit dose medications
   iv. Polypharmacy
   v. Patient counselling
   vi. Hospital formulary
b. How drug abuse is treated? Explain.
c. What advice will you give as a pharmacist to a patient taking (any *four*)
   i. Phenolphthalein
   ii. Antacid tablets
   iii. Amoxycillin
   iv. Emulsion and suspensions
   v. MAO inhibitor

d. 1. Define ADR. Classify ADR.
   2. Write normal values for (any four)
      i. W.B.C. Count
      ii. Sp. gr. of urine
      iii. Serum cholesterol
      iv. Haemoglobin—Male
      v. ESR

e. Distinguish between small volume parenterals and large volume parenterals.

Q 2. Answer any *three* of the following:

a. Classify hospitals giving one example of each type on the basis of:
   i. Size
   ii. Private ownership

b. Describe how physical properties of drug affect its bioavailability.

c. i. Differentiate between drug addiction and rug habituation.
   ii. Mention any four abilities that required for a hospital pharmacist.

d. Draw a labelled diagram and write uses of:
   i. Foley's Balloon catheter
   ii. Lane's tissue forceps

e. Define non-sterile manufacturing of drug. Write note on bulk concentrates.

Q 3. Answer any *three* of the following:

a. 1. Give an organisation chart of typical hospital.
   2. Define:
      i. Bioavailability
      ii. Absolute bioavailability.

b. What re the symptoms of chronic poisoning due to lead? How such patient is treated?

c. Describe:
   i. Satellite pharmacies
   ii. DIB

d. Enlist different aspects to be noted while taking medication history of a patient.

e. What is the utility of computers in purchases and inventory control in hospitals/medical stores?

Q 4. Answer any *three* of the following:

a. Define hospital pharmacy. State its any six functions.

b. Name any four types of drug food interactions. Explain with example one pharmacodynamic drug interactions.

c. Give four examples of each
   i. Hospital equipment
   ii. Health accessories

d. Enlist withdrawal symptoms and treatment of alcoholism.
e. Describe:
   i. Ryle's tube and its uses
   ii. CT scanner

Q 5. Answer any *three* of the following:

a. 1. Define:
   i. Outpatient
   ii. Central sterile service
   2. Define poisons and classify them with one example from each class.
b. What is HEPA filter? Write different additives in parenteral preparation.
c. Write:
   i. Contents of hospital formulary
   ii. Pathophysiology of angina pectoris
d. Describe any two tests for absorbency for standardisation of absorbent cotton, I.P.
e. What do you mean by:
   i. Emulsion
   ii. Fortis
   iii. Haematuria
   iv. Hora somni

Q 6. Answer any *three* of the following:

a. Comment on health delivery system in India at state level.
b. Write signs and symptoms of epilepsy.
c. Give organisation of PTC and its five functions.
d. Define 'clinical pharmacy'. Draw a chart/diagram indicating 'prominent role of a clinical pharmacist' in hospital.
e. 1. Explain any four reasons for patient non-compliance.
   2. Describe any for points on which a clinical pharmacist can counsel the patient.

Winter Examination 2011

D Pharm Second Year

Hospital and Clinical Pharmacy

Q 1. Attempt any *eight* of the following:

a. Define following hospital terms:
   i. Hospital formulary
   ii. Out-patient

b. State meaning of following:
   i. Elixir ii. Carminative
c. Mention suitable method of sterilization:
   i. Eye ointment ii. Rubber hand gloves
d. Write specific advise to patient taking:
   i. MAO inhibitors
   ii. Spermicidal Jellies and cream.
e. Write normal values of
   i. ESR ii. Serum cholesterol
f. Write use of following health accessories:
   i. Cane ii. Walker
g. Write antidote for:
   i. Arsenic ii. Morphine
h. Explain following pharmacological terms:
   i. Hypersensitivity ii. Synergism
i. Define following dosage forms:
   i. Poultice ii. Emulsion
j. Write use of following surgical instruments:
   i. Aneurysm needle ii. Lumber puncture needle
k. Define following clinical terms:
   i. Patient compliance ii. Adverse drug reaction
l. Write application of following:
   i. X-ray machine
   ii. Ryle's tube

Q 2. Answer any *four* of the following:

a. Define term drug abuse. How drug addicts are treated? Explain.
b. Give the organization chart of hospital.
c. Define DIC. Write sources of drug information.
d. Elaborate role of clinical pharmacist in developing country.
e. Write pathophysiology of hypertension.
f. Discuss any six objectives of hospital pharmacy.

Q 3. Answer any *four* of the following:

a. Write dispensing of medication to out patient.
b. Define patient counselling. Explain three role of pharmacist in patent counselling.
c. Explain one predictable ADRs with suitable examples.
d. Discuss two factors which governs the decision of manufacturing in hospital pharmacy.
e. Write any four guiding principle while using hospital formulary.
f. Classify poisons with examples.

Q 4. Answer any *four* of the following:

a. Write role of administrator in hospital.
b. Describe signs and symptoms of epilepsy.
c. Explain drug-food interaction with three examples.
d. How computer help in medication monitoring? Explain.
e. Define unit dose medication. Write benefits of unit dose dispensing.
f. Write withdrawl symptoms of alcohol and its treatment.

Q 5. Answer any *four* of the following:

a. Mention abilities of the chief hospital pharmacist. Explain any one of them.
b. Write symptoms of acute arsenic poisoning and treatment of it.
c. Write difference between drug addiction and drug habituation.
d. Give an account of medication history of a patient.
e. Define ADR. Write causes of ADR.
f. Explain term bandage. Describe two examples of bandages with its use.

Q 6. Attempt any *four* of the following:

a. Describe any two pharmaceutical factors affecting bioavailability of drugs.
b. Write location and layout of hospital pharmacy
c. Explain one pharmacodynamic drug interaction with example.
d. What is HEPA filter? Describe its working.
e. Write pathophysiology of diabetes mellitus.
f. Write role of PTC in drug safety in hospital.

Summer Examination 2012

D Pharm Second Year

Hospital and Clinical Pharmacy

Q 1. Solve any *eight*:

a. Define (any *two*):
   i. Hospital
   ii. Hospital pharmacy
   iii. Clinical pharmacy
b. Mention suitable method for sterilization (any *two*):
   i. Hand gloves
   ii. Sutures
   iii. Glassware
c. Give the normal values (any *two*):
   i. Blood cholesterol
   ii. Sperm count
   iii. Erythrocytes

d. Mention the doses of the following:
   i. Dimercaprol
   ii. EDTA
e. Translate following terms in English (any *two*):
   i. Collyrium
   ii. Pasta
   iii. Dolore urgente
f. Give the uses of (any *two*):
   i. CT scanner
   ii. Ultrasound sonography
   iii. Arthroscope
g. What is first pass effect?
h. What these abbreviations stand for (any *two*)?
   i. IAI
   ii. BAL
   iii. ECG
i. What is elite pharmacy?
j. Name two preservatives used in parenteral preparations.
k. Name four quality control tests for parenterals.
l. What is drug information bulletin?

Q 2. Solve any *four*:

a. Classify hospitals on clinical basis.
b. What is hospital formulary system?
c. What are the qualities of pharmacist required to run DIS?
d. Describe the factors affecting economy of hospital.
e. What is the role of Nursing department in a hospital?
f. Give three methods of estimating demand.

Q 3. Solve any *four*:

a. Enlist the name of standards prescribed by IP for absorbency of absorbent cotton. Describe it.
b. Describe the application of computers in pharmacy.
c. Explain the factors affecting make or buy decision in hospital manufacturing.
d. What re surgical instruments? Give uses of following instruments:
   i. Haemostatic forcep
   ii. Scalpel
e. What is PTC? Give the role of PTC in drug safety.
f. State the meaning of:
   i. Cold
   ii. Cool
   iii. Freeze

Q 4. Solve any *four*:

a. Define patient-compliance and patient non-compliance. Give two reasons for patient non-compliance.
b. Define and classify ADR.
c. What is clinical pharmacy? Give the responsibilities of clinical pharmacist regarding use of therapeutic drugs.
d. Define the following terms:
   i. Etiology
   ii. Manifestation
   iii. Pathogenesis
e. Give the meaning of following terms:
   i. Apnoea
   ii. Eosinophilia
   iii. Ischaemia
f. What is antidote? Give the formula and uses of universal antidote.

Q 5. Solve any *four*:

a. Define:
   i. Idiosyncracy
   ii. Teratogenicity
   iii. Phocomelia
b. Give the general procedure for treatment of poisoning.
c. Enlist various factors which affect bioavailability of drug. Describe pharmaceutical factors.
d. What is the role of pharmacist in patient counselling?
e. State the conditions which leads to heart failure. Give the sings and symptoms of CHF.
f. Define:
   i. Bioavailability
   ii. Bioequivalence
   iii. Relative bioavailability

Q 6. Solve any *four*:

a. Name various methods for sterilization. Write the principle involved in Autoclave.
b. Describe floor stock system. Give its advantages and disadvantages.
c. Give the composition and function of PTC.
d. What advice a pharmacist should offer to the patient for following drugs (any *two*)?
   i. MAO-inhibitors
   ii. Chewable antacid tablet
   iii. Salicylates

e. Explain drug interactions (any *two*):
   i. Folic acid and phenytoin
   ii. Warfarin and phenobarbitone
   iii. Aspirin and penicillin
f. Differentiate between drug addiction and rug habituation.

Winter Examination 2012

D Pharm Second Year

Hospital and Clinical Pharmacy

Q 1. Answer any *eight*:

a. Define:
   i. Drug abuse
   ii. Hospital
b. What is HEPA filter?
c. What do you mean by:
   i. Emulsion
   ii. Hora Somni
d. Give the normal values of:
   i. Specific gravity of urine.
   ii. Blood cholesterol.
e. Give any two reasons for patient non-compliance.
f. What is Lane's tissue forcep?
g. What is:
   i. Chemical equivalence
   ii. Biological equivalence
h. Define the terms referred and ambulatory patient.
i. What are teratogens? Give one example.
j. What is BAL? Mention its use.
k. Give the composition of universal antidote.
l. Explain the constitution of PTC.

Q 2. Answer any *four*:

a. Give the reasons of adverse drug reactions.
b. What advice you will give as a pharmacist to a patient taking:
   i. MAO inhibitors
   ii. Antacid tablets
   iii. Diazepam
c. Write the uses of:
   i. Scalpel
   ii. ECG machine
   iii. Foley's catheter

d. Discuss about the objectives of hospital pharmacy.
e. Describe the health delivery system in India.
f. Differentiate between drug addiction and drug habituation.

Q 3. Answer any *four*:

a. Give any three functions of PTC
b. What are the merits of unit dose dispensing?
c. Discuss in brief about drug and food interaction.
d. Discuss any two examples of diuretic drug interactions.
e. Give the signs ad symptoms of rheumatoid arthritis.
f. Enlist the equipment needed for the preparation of parenterals.

Q 4. Answer any *four*:

a. What is idiosyncrasy and allergy?
b. Discuss in brief, how the medication history is taken.
c. How absorbent cotton wool is evaluated as per IP?
d. Discuss the clinical significance of ESR.
e. Write the procedure adopted by hospital pharmacist to procure drugs.
f. What is bed side pharmacy? Give its importance.

Q 5. Answer any *four*:

a. Mention the uses of following:
   i. CT scanner
   ii. Lithotripsy
   iii. Haemostatic forceps
b. Translate into English:
   i. SOS
   ii. Gutta
   iii. qid
c. Write the applications of computers in retail pharmacy.
d. Write the primary and secondary sources of drug information bulletin.
e. Discuss three physiological factors which affect bioavailability.
f. Discuss about the general steps involved in the treatment of poisoning.

Q 6. Answer any *four*:

a. Discuss about the scope of clinical pharmacy.
b. State the meaning of:
   i. Emetics
   ii. Carminatives
   iii. Anaemia
   iv. Insomnia

c. Discuss in brief about hospital formulary.
d. Classify the hospitals on four different basis.
e. Discuss in brief about hallucinogens.
f. What is tuberculosis? Write its pathophysiology, signs and symptoms.

Summer Examination 2013

D Pharm Second Year

Hospital and Clinical Pharmacy

Q 1. Attempt the following:

a. Define any four of the following
   i. Bioavailability.
   ii. Unit dose dispensing
   iii. Teratogenicity
   iv. Hallucinogen
   v. Non-sterile manufacturing
   vi. Pharmacy therapeutic committee.

b. Answer any two of the following:
   i. Give the requirement of pharmacist in hospital as per the bed capacity.
   ii. What are crepe bandages?
   iii. Composition and use of universal antidote.

c. Explain any two of the following:
   i. Anaphylaxis
   ii. Chronic poisoning
   iii. C.T. scanner

d. State the meaning of any four of following:
   i. Tranquilizers
   ii. Carminatives
   iii. Necrosis
   iv. Anorexia
   v. Cholagogue

e. What is megaloblastic and haemolytic anemia? Give example of drugs causing these anemia.

Q 2. Attempt any *three* of the following:

a. Describe procedure of dispensing of non-charge floor stock drugs in hospital.
b. Give the various administrative pattern of CSSD.
c. What is patient counselling? Write factors responsible for non-compliance.
d. Classify pharmacokinetic drug interaction with examples.
e. Define bioequivalence. What is first (1st) pass effect?

Q 3. Attempt any *three* of the following:

a. Define and give reason for ADR.
b. Describe symptoms and treatment for chronic lead poisoning.
c. How drugs are added and deleted in hospital formulary?
d. Define hospital and give its function.
e. Name the different equipment required for tablet manufacturing

Q 4. Attempt any *three* of the following:

a. Define physiological parameters. Write normal values of:
   i. Blood cholesterol
   ii. DLC.
b. Describe BAL as an antidote in poisoning.
c. Write a note on drug information retrieval by computers.
d. What are surgical dressings? Classify surgical adhesive tapes.
e. Who is an outpatient? Classify any two types of outpatient.

Q 5. Attempt any *three* of the following:

a. Define formulary and give reasons for need of it.
b. Describe pathophysiology of hepatitis.
c. Differentiate between psychological and physical drug dependence.
d. What is clinical pharmacy and give its objectives?
e. Draw floor plan of sterile product area.

Q 6. Attempt any *three* of the following:

a. Explain how pka, partition coefficient and gastric transit time affect bioavailability.
b. What are the technical and administrative abilities required for hospital pharmacist?
c. Give conditions to be fulfilled by all parenterals.
d. Comment on the different sources of drug information.
e. Explain food drug interactions with examples.

Winter Examination 2013

D Pharm Second Year

Hospital and Clinical Pharmacy

Q 1. Attempt the following:

a. Define the following: (Any *two*)
   i. Drug abuse
   ii. Hospital
   iii. Etiology
   iv. Clinical pharmacy
b. Give normal values with significance:
   i. RBC count
   ii. ESR

c. Translate into English: (Any *four*)

i. Tussis | ii. Unus
iii. Bis in die | iv. Dandus
v. Capiondus | vi. Urgenti

d. State the meaning of:

i. Emetics | ii. Carminative
iii. Anorexia | iv. Purgative

e. Write the one example of each poison:

i. Corrosive | ii. Organic
iii. Irritant | iv. Inorganic

Q 2. Attempt any *three*:

a. Give importance of nursing services and medical record services in hospital.
b. What is hospital formulary? Give guideline principles for preparation of hospital formulary.
c. Name various methods of sterilization. Write the principle involved in autoclaving.
d. Classify the hospital in the basis of ownership.
e. Give composition and function of PTC.

Q 3. Attempt any *three*:

a. What do you means by drug induced disease? Give various drug induced diseases.
b. Define the patient compliance. Give six factors affecting compliance.
c. Give requirement for location and layout for outpatient pharmacy.
d. Explain factors influencing make or buy decision in hospital. What are different methods of estimation of demands?
e. Enumerate factors affecting bio-availability of drugs. What is bio-equivalence?

Q 4. Attempt any *three*:

a. Classify ADR with examples.
b. State pathophysiology, sing and symptoms of any one disease.
   i. Peptic ulcer
   ii. Heart attack
c. Explain the role of computer in purchase and inventory control in hospital.
d. Define non-sterile manufacturing. What are requirements for tablet?
e. Give location and layout of central sterile room or sterile manufacturing area.

Q 5. Attempt any *three*:

a. Name any 4-surgical dressing. Give standards for absorbent cotton wool IP.

b. Discuss the health delivery system in India.

c. Give qualification and abilities required for running drug information center. What drug information bulletin?

d. What are withdrawal symptoms of alcohol and write treatment for it.

e. Define Drug interaction. Explain pharmacokinetic drug interaction with example.

Q 6. Attempt any *three*:

a. Give any four drugs which cause addition. How drug abuse treated?

b. Give classification of poison. What are steps involved in general treatment of poison?

c. Discuss the floor stock system with merits and demerits.

d. Write short notes on:
   i. Prepackaging
   ii. Benefits of UDD system

e. Enlist eight functions of hospital.

Winter Examination 2014

D Pharm Second Year

Hospital and Clinical Pharmacy

Q 1. Attempt any *five* of the following:

a. Give normal values and significance of any *two*

i. Blood cholesterol	ii. ESR
iii. Sperm count	

b. What advice must be given to the patient using any *four*

i. MAO inhibitors	ii. Aspirin
iii. Diazepam	iv. Ampicillin
v. Phenytoin	vi. Boric acid

c. Write one example of each of the following poison:

i. Corrosive	ii. Organic
iii. Inorganic	iv. Cardiac

d. Define the following:

i. Teratogenicity	ii. Addison's disease
iii. Choleretics	iv. Drug abuse

e. Translate into English:

i. Dandus	ii. Semel in die
iii. Tussis	iv. Charta

f. Write the use of following: (Any *four*)
   i. ECG machines
   ii. CT scanners
   iii. Doppler echocardiography
   iv. Sphygmomanometer
   v. Ultrasound sonography
   vi. Magnetic resonance imaging (MRI)

g. Write the meaning of following abbreviations:
   i. LAL ii. TPN
   iii. SVP iv. HEPA

Q 2. Attempt any *three* of the following:

a. Define hospital. Write the functions of hospital.
b. Explain the process of dispensing drugs to outpatients in a typical hospital.
c. Explain the factors affecting make or buy decision in hospital manufacturing.
d. Define hospital pharmacy. State the objectives of hospital pharmacy.
e. Differentiate between drug addiction and drug habituation.

Q 3. Attempt any *three* of the following:

a. Define adverse drug reaction and write a note about Idiosyncrasy
b. Explain the role of computer in:
   i. Medication monitoring in hospital
   ii. Purchasing and inventory control in hospital.
c. Define:
   i. Bioavailability
   ii. Bioequivalence
   iii. Relative bioavailability
   iv. Absolute bioavailability
d. Define PTC. Describe role of PTC in drugs safety.
e. Define surgical dressings. Describe any three tests to be performed to evaluate absorbent cotton wool IP

Q 4. Attempt any *three* of the following:

a. Explain pathophysiology, signs and symptoms of 'Tuberculosis'.
b. Define 'Drug Information Bulletin'. Give the different sources of collecting drug information.
c. Define clinical pharmacy and describe its scope.
d. Explain the following drug interactions:
   i. Folic acid and phenytoin
   ii. Warfarin and phenobarbitone.
f. Define antidote. Give the formula and uses of universal antidote.

Q 5. Attempt any *three* of the following:

a. Define nonsterile manufacturing. Name the equipment required for manufacturing of tablets.
b. Discuss the guiding principles of 'Hospital Formulary System'.
c. Explain pathophysiology, signs and symptoms of 'peptic ulcer'.
d. What do you mean by centralized and decentralized purchase? Describe to whom the copies of purchase order are given and why?
e. Explain the uses of following:
   i. Aneurysm needle
   ii. Lithotripsy
   iii. Ryle's tube
   iv. Rubber catheter

Q 6. Attempt any *three* of the following:

a. Explain the terms:
   i. General patient
   ii. Referred patient
   iii. Emergency patient
   iv. Ambulatory patient.
b. Classify hospitals giving one examples of each type on the basis of:
   i. Size
   ii. Private ownership
c. Explain the mechanisms of pharmacodynamic drug interactions.
d. Describe any eight factors contributing to patient non-compliance.

Summer Examination 2015

D Pharm Second Year

Hospital and Clinical Pharmacy

Q 1. Attempt any *eight* of the following:

a. Define hospital pharmacy. Give its objectives.
b. What do you mean by SWF1 and WFI?
c. Define PTC. Give its composition.
d. What is hospital formulary? Give its need.
e. Give ideal properties of surgical dressing.
f. Give any two applications of computer.
g. What advice will you give to patients about following drugs:
   i. Antacid tablet
   ii. Diazepam
h. Define allergy, antidote.
i. Give normal physiological value of
   i. Blood cholesterol
   ii. ESR
j. Define:
   i. Adverse drug reaction
   ii. Idiosyncracy
k. What is universal antidote ? Give its composition.
l. Define drug dependence and drug abuse.

Q 2. Attempt any *four* of the following:

a. Draw and explain layout of central sterile services.
b. Give functions and scope of PTC.
c. Explain role of pharmacist in patient counselling.
d. Define Angina Pectoris. Give its pathophysiology.
e. Define clinical pharmacy. Give services of clinical pharmacist.
f. Define Bioavailability. Give factors affecting on it.

Q 3. Attempt any *four* of the following:

a. Define hospital. Give its functions.
b. What is satellite pharmacy service? Give its location and advantages.
c. Give uses of the following :
   i. CT scan
   ii. Surgical gloves
   iii. Autoclave
d. Define patient non-compliance. Explain role of pharmacist in it.
e. What is drug food interaction? Explain with example.
f. Define poison. Give its classification.

Q 4. Attempt any *four* of the following:

a. Explain responsibilities of hospital pharmacist in relation to patient care.
b. Enlist methods of drug distribution in hospital. Give advantages and disadvantages of mobile dispensing unit.
c. Explain the importance of computer in inventory control.
d. Give pathophysiology and manifestation of rheumatoid arthritis.
e. Define ADR. Give its classification.
f. Describe mechanism of drug absorption.

Q 5. Attempt any *four* of the following:

a. Give requirement and abilities required for hospital pharmacist.
b. Give objectives of inventory control. Explain procedure of purchasing.
c. Write a note on preparation of formulary.
d. What is DIB? Give its importance.
e. Differentiate between drug addiction and drug habitation.
f. Give dose of following:
   i. BAL
   ii. EDTA
   iii. Penicillamine

Q 6. Attempt any *four* of the following:

a. Explain the evaluation parameters of parenterals.
b. Explain the different sources of drug information.

c. Define surgical dressing. Give monograph of cotton.
d. What is peptic ulcer? Give its types and pathophysiology.
e. Give clinical significance of following:
   i. Clotting time   ii. B.P.
f. What is acute poisoning? Give general treatment of poisoning.

Winter Examination 2015

D Pharm Second Year

Hospital and Clinical Pharmacy

Q 1. Attempt any *ten* of the following:

a. Define hospital and floor-stock.
b. Write four types of forceps.
c. Define (any **two**):
   i. Drug abuse   ii. Pyrogen
   iii. Antidote
d. Explain (any **two**):
   i. Bioequivalence   ii. Hallucinogen
   iii. Lithotripsy
e. Write one example of corrosive and mechanical poison.
f. Write about anaphylaxis or idiosyncracy.
g. Write result of drug interaction: (any **two**)
   i. Warfarin along with salicylates
   ii. Rifampicin along with oral contraceptives
   iii. Alcohol with CNS depressant
   iv. Digitalis glycosides along with antacid.
h. What advice should be given to patient who takes: (any **two**)
   i. Antidiabetic drug   ii. Ampicillin
   iii. Tetracycline   iv. Diazepam
i. Write normal values and significance of (any **two**)
   i. Haemoglobin   ii. Blood pressure
   iii. WBC   iv. Blood sugar
j. Translate into English: (any **four**)
   i. Cataplasm   ii. Collyr
   iii. Garg   iv. Ung
   v. Unus   vi. Tussis
k. Write names of four quality control tests performed on parenterals or tablets.
l. What is meaning of the following: (any **four**)
   i. ICU   ii. CCF
   iii. KUB   iv. BBB
   v. HRT   vi. UTI

Q 2. Attempt any *three* of the following:

a. Define and write functions of hospital pharmacy.
b. Describe functions of hospital administrator.
c. Write purpose, principles and contents of medical record.
d. Classify hospitals on the basis of ownership.
e. Draw and describe flow chart of patients in hospital.

Q 3. Attempt any *three* of the following:

a. Describe location and layout of out patient dispensary.
b. How pre-packaging is carried out? What are its benefits?
c. What are charge floor-stock drugs? What are methods to dispense the drugs?
d. What is central service? Write three administrative patterns of central service.
e. Explain how purchase order is prepared and distributed.

Q 4. Attempt any *three* of the following:

a. What is laminar flow? Write about laminar flow bench with diagram.
b. Describe layout of sterite products area with diagram.
c. Write composition, functions of PTC. What is role of PTC in ADR?
d. What is hospital formulary? What are contents of hospital formulary?
e. What qualities should be required for the pharmacist to run drug information services?

Q 5. Attempt any *three* of the following:

a. Mention four categories of surgical dressings and mention two tests to evaluate absorbent cotton.
b. How computers are useful to maintain records in hospital?
c. Write sources of drug information.
d. Define clinical pharmacy. Write functions of clinical pharmacist.
e. Describe procurement or purchase procedure step by step.

Q 6. Attempt any *three* of the following:

a. What is patient compliance? Which instructions should be given by pharmacist to patient to improve compliance?
b. Define and classify adverse drug reaction.
c. Define teratogen. Describe teratogenicity.
d. Define bioavailability. Write factors affecting unavailability. Discuss physical factors which affect it.
e. Write pathophysiology, signs and symptoms and complications of diabetes or arthritis.

Summer Examination 2016

D Pharm Second Year

Hospital and Clinical Pharmacy

Q 1. Attempt the following:

a. Define the following: (any **four**)

i. Hospital pharmacy
ii. Drug information service
iii. Patient compliance
iv. Drug interaction
v. Hospital formulary

b. What advice will you give to the patient taking: (any **four**)

i. Diazepam
ii. Tetracycline
iii. Phenolphthalein
iv. MAO inhibitors
v. Boric acid

c. Give normal values of: (any **four**)

i. Heart rate
ii. RBC
iii. ESR
iv. Sperm count
v. Blood sugar

d. Translate into English: (any **four**)

i. Guttae
ii. Bis in die
iii. Nebula
iv. Omni nocte
v. Collutorium

e. Explain the following: (any **four**)

i. Lithotripsy
ii. Drug habituation
iii. Idiosyncrasy
iv. PTC and drug safety
v. Triple roller ointment mill

Q 2. Attempt any *three* of the following:

a. Define modem hospital and write its functions.
b. Explain the abilities and competence required for a hospital pharmacist.
c. Explain receipt and issue system in out-patient dispensing.
d. Define clinical pharmacy and describe its scope.
e. Write the 'consequences of non-compliance'.

Q 3. Attempt any *three* of the following:

a. Write pathophysiology, signs and symptoms of 'myocardial Infarction' or 'rheumatoid arthritis'.
b. Explain 'drug-food interaction'.
c. Define unit dose dispensing. Write its benefits.
d. Define central services. Give various administrative patterns of central services.
e. Discuss four important factors governing make or buy decision.

Q 4. Attempt any *three* of the following:

a. Name and explain the various additives used in the parenteral formulation.
b. Describe the procurement or purchase procedure step-by-step.
c. Define adverse drug reaction. Explain the various reasons for adverse reactions.
d. Classify poisons with examples.
e. Give medical complications, withdrawal symptoms and treatment of alcoholism.

Q 5. Attempt any *three* of the following:

a. What is bioavailability? Discuss physiological factors affecting bioavailability of drugs.
b. What are antidotes ? Classify them with examples.
c. Write the guiding principles while using a hospital formulary.
d. Write any four tests to evaluate 'absorbent cotton wool IP.
e. Explain the use of computers in purchasing and inventory control.

Q 6. Attempt any *three* of the following:

a. Give a short account of hospitals classified on the basis of size.
b. Explain the following:
   i. Haematinics
   ii. Anaesthetics
   iii. Cholagogues
   iv. Tranquilizers
c. Explain the 'floor stock system'.
d. Explain the role of pharmacist in monitoring adverse drug reactions.
e. Explain 'pyrogen testing'.

Winter Examination 2016

D Pharm Second Year

Hospital and Clinical Pharmacy

Q 1. Solve any *eight* of the following:

a. Define the following terms: (any **one**)
   i. Modern hospital
   ii. Clinical pharmacy
   iii. Bioavailability
b. Give the normal values of: (any **four**)
   i. Haemoglobin % in females
   ii. Normal blood sugar
   iii. Clotting time of blood
   iv. Specific gravity of urine

v. Sperm count
vi. ESR in males and females

c. What advice must be given to patients while using following drugs: (any **two**)
   i. Antacid tablets   ii. Boric acid
   iii. Antidiabetics   iv. Diphenhydramine
d. State the meanings of: (any **one**)
   i. Drug abuse   ii. Bioequivalence
e. List the factors affecting bioavailability of drugs.
f. Draw the flowchart for out-patients in a typical hospital.
g. What are the benefits of unit dose dispensing.
h. Name and draw different needles used in a surgical hospital.
i. Name two databases available for computerized drug information retrieval.
j. List two objectives for taking medication history of patients.
k. Write an example of each of the following poisons:
   i. Corrosives   ii. Irritants
   iii. Organic   iv. Inorganic
l. Write the antidotes for: (any **two**)
   i. Physostigmine   ii. Pentazocine
   iii. Ethylene glycol   iv. Quinidine

Q 2. Solve any *four* of the following:

a. What are the objectives of hospital pharmacy?
b. List the technical abilities required for hospital pharmacist.
c. Define a modern hospital and classify hospitals clinically.
d. What are the purposes, principles and importance of medical records in a hospital?
e. Define general out-patient. Write about 10 lines on location and layout of OPD.
f. Explain the concept of clinical pharmacy (in about **10** lines).

Q 3. Solve any *four* of the following:

a. Explain the pre-packing activity in a hospital (in about **10** lines).
b. Explain the receipt and issue system of medicines in an OPD.
c. How are the charged stock drugs selected and dispensed to in-patients of a hospital?
d. Explain the "bedside pharmacy" in a hospital.
e. Where should the CSSD department be located in a hospital? Which are the areas in which the manpower of this department should be trained?
f. List and explain the economic factors affecting make or buy decision of medicines in a hospital.

Q 4. Solve any *four* of the following:

a. List the aseptic work precautions for working in a sterile area.
b. List the properties for parenteral products. How is a parenteral formula developed?
c. Which are the equipments for manufacture of pills and compressed tablets as per drugs and cosmetics act and rules?
d. When and how should a re-order be placed for materials in a hospital?
e. What are the functions of PTC? What is its role in drug safety?
f. List the various surgical dressings? How is absorbent cotton prepared and identified?

Q 5. Solve any *four* of the following:

a. What are the consequences of non-compliance by patients to prescription?
b. Write 5 lines on: (any **two**)
   i. Antidiuretic hormone
   ii. Vaccines
   iii. Immunity
c. Define adverse drug reactions. What are the causes of ADR?
d. Explain the pathophysiology of gastric ulcer.
e. What is hospital formulary? Give the guiding principles for preparing hospital formulary.
f. Explain how purchase order is prepared.

Q 6. Solve any *four* of the following:

a. Define drug interactions. Give various mechanisms of drug interaction with example of each.
b. How do pharmaceutical factors affect bioavailability of drugs?
c. What is teratogenicity? Explain in 10 lines with its effects.
d. Explain the principle and working of an "autoclave".
e. What are the signs and symptoms of rheumatoid arthritis?
f. Classify poisons. What are the steps involved in general treatment of poisoning?

Summer Examination 2017

D Pharm Second Year

Hospital and Clinical Pharmacy

Q 1. Solve any *eight* of the following:

a. Define: (any **two**)
   i. ADR
   ii. Patient compliance
   iii. Hospital pharmacy

b. Give the normal values of: (any **two**)
   i. Creatinine ii. Blood cholesterol
   iii. Sperm count
c. Translate following terms in English: (any **two**)
   i. Utendus ii. Guttae
   iii. Omni mane
d. Give the uses of: (any **two**)
   i. ECG ii. Aneurysm needle
   iii. Ryle's tube
e. Explain term first pass effect.
f. Define hallucinogen. Write effects of LSD.
g. Write the requirement of number of pharmacists in a hospital pharmacy.
h. What are Elite hospitals?
i. Give the objectives of inventory control.
j. What advice must be given to the patient using: (any **two**)
   i. Tetracycline ii. Bisacodyl
   iii. Phenytoin
k. What is BAL? Mention its use.
l. Distinguish between small volume parenterals and large volume parenterals.

Q 2. Solve any *four* of the following:

a. Define clinical pharmacy. Draw a chart/diagram indicating role of clinical pharmacist in the hospital.
b. State the objectives of hospital pharmacy.
c. Write signs, symptoms and treatment of opium poisoning.
d. Write the uses of:
   i. Crepe bandage
   ii. Plaster of paris bandage
   iii. Zinc paste bandage
e. Give the methods of estimating demand of product in hospital.
f. Enumerate the reasons for patient non-compliance.

Q 3. Solve any *four* of the following:

a. Classify hospital according to clinical parameters with examples.
b. Give the meaning of following terms: (any **three**)
   i. Emetics ii. Cholagogue
   iii. Gout iv. Hypoxia
e. Explain any three factors affecting bioavailability.
d. Explain with examples drug-food interactions.
e. Describe the role of PTC in drug safety.
f. What is rheumatoid arthritis? Describe the pathophysiology of RA.

Q 4. Solve any *four* of the following:

a. Define parenterals. Describe the following test for evaluation of parenteral solution: Sterility test or pyrogen test.
b. How drug abuse is treated?
c. Write sources of collection of drug information at DIC.
d. Explain the use of computer in inventory control in hospital pharmacy.
e. Explain term: 'Teratogen. Give any two examples of teratogenic drugs alongwith its teratogenic effects.
f. What is (i) Lithotripsy, (ii) Lane's tissue forcep, (iii) MRI?

Q 5. Solve any *four* of the following:

a. Describe the processing of parenterals.
b. Write pathophysiology of heart attack. Write the clinical manifestations of it.
c. What is the role of nursing department in hospitals?
d. Discuss the guiding principles of hospital formulary system.
e. List the withdrawal symptoms and write treatment of morphine dependence.
f. Explain terms: (any **three**)
   i. Bioavailability
   ii. Relative bioavailability
   iii. Clinical equivalence
   iv. Therapeutic equivalence

Q 6. Solve any *four* of the following:

a. Define drug interaction. Explain what will happen when following drug administered together:
   i. Folic acid with phenytoin
   ii. Digitalis with diuretics
   iii. Alcohol with disulfiram
b. Draw the diagram of IV set. Describe the functions of its components.
c. Write a note on:
   i. DIB
   ii. Satellite pharmacy
d. Discuss economic factors governing the manufacture and purchase decision in production in hospital pharmacy.
e. Write the dose and uses of dimercaprol and desferrioxamine in toxicology.
f. How is dispensing of charged floor stock carried out? Write any two advantages and disadvantages of complete floor stock system.